# EATING PROMISCUOUSLY

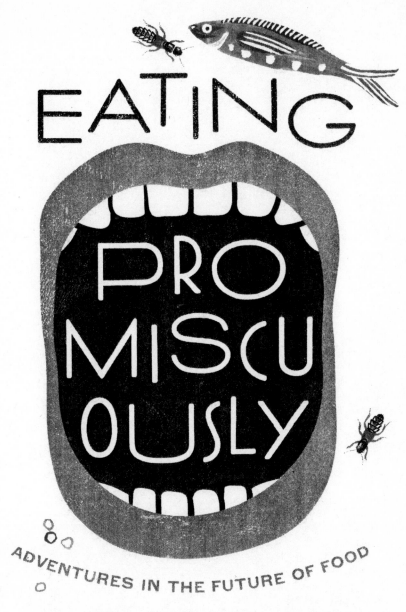

# EATING PRO MISCU OUSLY

ADVENTURES IN THE FUTURE OF FOOD

## JAMES MCWILLIAMS

COUNTERPOINT

BERKELEY

Library of Congress Cataloging-in-Publication Data Is Available.


Cover design by Faceout Studio
Interior design by Tabitha Lahr

ISBN 978-1-61902-735-0

COUNTERPOINT
2560 Ninth Street, Suite 318
Berkeley, CA 94710
www.counterpointpress.com

Printed in the United States of America
Distributed by Publishers Group West

10 9 8 7 6 5 4 3 2 1

Dedication: TK

# CONTENTS

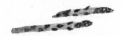

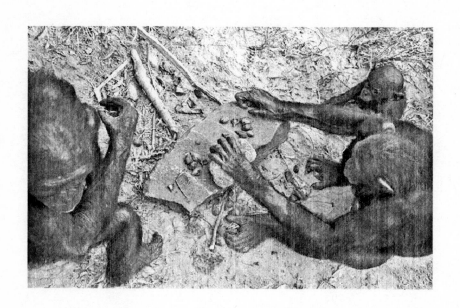

# The Bonobo Diet

> *"Your discovery, as best as I can determine, is that there is an*
> *alternative which no one has hit upon."*
>
> —WALKER PERCY, *The Moviegoer*

Human beings have been eating food for almost 3 million years. But we've only been practicing agriculture—the act of forcing plants and animals to stay in one place—for about the last 12,000. That's only .02 percent of our total existence. Industrial agriculture, the kind of farming that "feeds the world," has been around for about 100 years, thus stretching that .02 percent to .000025 percent. That's decimal dust.

The way we eat today is brand new—a recent thunderbolt of human experimentation with you and me as the subjects. Not only is it new; it's barely a distant echo of anything that came before. Given its late arrival, and given its lack of precedent, agriculture by its nature raises an interesting question: Why should we think we got it right the first time around? Given the process of trial and error behind every other example of human progress, who would ever believe we'd succeed on the first shot?

This book opens with the claim that we didn't. In fact, it assumes we thoroughly screwed it up. This assessment holds true not just for the last century—when our agricultural sins intensified to the point that we finally took notice—but for the entire ongoing human effort to domesticate plants and animals for food. The food system isn't broken—it was never fixed.

Locate blame where you see fit, but agricultural development has been a largely unthinking decision made by hundreds of generations through billions of ad-hoc choices about how to secure a consistent supply of food. There's no single person, corporation, politician, advertising executive, or USDA official to condemn for what we now reap as food. Still, it's a reality we must live with every time we sit at the table. The collective decision to practice the sort of agriculture we practice—clear space, plant seeds, tend plants, harvest, feed most of it to animals, repeat—has reduced something as necessary to human life as eating to a handful of nutritionally depleted foods. All the while it has asked us to accept the situation as normal.

I'm hardly the first person to make this case. When it comes to the task of feeding ourselves, according to Jared Diamond, author of *Collapse,* we went off the rails about 10,000 years ago. He has called agriculture "the worst mistake in the history of the human race," the leading source of "malnutrition, starvation, and epidemic diseases," and the underlying reason for such troubles as ecological devastation, "deep class divisions," and exploitative power hierarchies. Another critic, Richard Manning, develops a similar argument in *Against the Grain: How Agriculture Hijacked Civilization.* He contends that from the outset human farmers have proven poorly equipped "to deal with the abundance" generated by agriculture. As he understands it, agriculture per se leads to a spew of food that increasingly ruins human health (even if we are living longer lives) while destroying the natural environment. Victor Davis Hanson, a former California raisin farmer turned classics professor, furthers the anti-agriculture missive in *Fields without Dreams*, arguing that farming, when you get down to it, is "a foolhardly thing to do."

If prominent thinkers have questioned the nature of agriculture, reformers seeking solutions have yet to heed the message. Instead, they've worked safely within the confines of the established agricultural regime that Diamond and his fellow critics denounce. The progressive solutions we currently entertain—eat local, eat organic, eat from small farms, eat whole foods, eat what grandma ate—are, in their small contexts, sensible steps to take. But they're no more than Band-Aid solutions. They assume, quite incorrectly, that agriculture is a habit that once was, and once again can be, consistent with the cycles of nature. They look back, in many ways, to a past that never existed. This is no way to revolutionize how we eat.

The moral weight invested in these popular alternatives makes it seem as if the most important food issue we face today is simply about making better choices within an existing range of options (or just bringing smaller versions of the old options into existence). Eating "food with integrity"—Chipotle's clever slogan—sourced from local farmers who raise their own hogs has prevented us from fundamentally rethinking the choices themselves. The fact that Chipotle—a glorified fast food hub that has recently suffered from a spate of tainted food products—has come to symbolize reform says a lot about how low the bar for food reform has been set.

Then there's the propaganda. A veritable cottage industry of nostalgic agrarian literature—a trend that has nearly turned farming into poetry—has clogged bookstore shelves with bucolic mythologies centered on the pre-industrial farmer. He has become a virtuous figure working in tandem with nature to bring us a pesticide-free, family-farm-strengthening, value- enhancing cornucopia. This genre—which sustains the local, organic, and "slow" alternative to industrial farming—has seduced us through a kind of agrarian pornography that ultimately glorifies the system that oppresses us. Bolder thinking is required.

By assuming that, when it comes to agriculture, we (or at least our ancestors) failed on the first attempt, and by dismissing the present alternatives as inadequate (however romantically the alternatives are presented), this book suggests a different starting point for saving our food system. Admittedly, it's a thought experiment—and possibly a fantastic one But it has the benefit of freeing our imagination to think in more ambitious terms: What if we could wipe the slate clean and, given what we now know, imagine a radically new way for humans to eat?

*What if we could start over?*

Reengineer the system. Sit with the notion a bit and it becomes a liberating idea. It frees us to think far beyond where we've ventured before, at least when it comes to reforming food and agriculture. It permits us to pursue improbable but critical "what if" thoughts without getting bogged down by practicalities, much less the predictable resistance, compromises, and political contestations that follow most agricultural proposals. It allows us to drop out, tune in, and dream a little.

I realize that this kind of gambit might seem escapist, superfluous, or even a little naïve. But it's none of these things. In fact, it's perfectly consistent with the deeper nature of long-term human behavior. It honors how human progress—especially when it comes to something so elemental to life such as food—is ultimately based on getting it wrong before we get it right.

Ideally, the result of Agriculture Plan B would be a global food system that's accessible, flexible, abundant, sustainable, healthy, humane, and resourceful. But most importantly, more than any other feature, it would be *diverse*. I stress "diverse" because all the other beneficial qualities would, I believe, naturally follow from a future food system that generates more varieties of more foods to directly consume rather than, as is now the case, greater volumes of the same old stuff, most of which is grown to feed animals.

This bemoaning of today's culinary monotony may sound counterintuitive. Calorically speaking, there's more food being produced now than at any other point in human history.[1] Walk through a grocery store in an industrialized nation (food deserts notwithstanding) and you'll encounter a cornucopia of options that ostensibly allows consumers to tailor food decisions to our most capricious cravings.

And the outcome is, in the short term, something of a pleasure fest. Want a gluten free, low-fat, non-GMO cookie with dairy-free chocolate chips? You got it. Want it to be super-sized and without artificial flavors? No problem. Ordering a drink in Starbucks these days practically requires being fluent in a foreign language ("grande skinny half-caf-

---

1. http://www.worldhunger.org/2015-world-hunger-and-poverty-facts-and-statistics/

latte"?). But all the terminology reflects, as with the food system itself, variations on a single theme. Never have we had so much food and so many apparent choices at our fingertips. Never have we been so blessed with such abundance. You might reasonably ask: why would anyone take issue with this progress?

The embarrassment of riches is, for all its flash, a delusion. The options we encounter on the shelves of a first-world grocery store might appear to represent a dazzling array of culinary diversity. But what we're actually encountering are aisles upon aisles—and menus upon menus—of food manufactured from the same handful of uninspired ingredients: starch, sugar, soy, corn, and fat. Even among non-processed foods there's minimal diversity. There are 7,500 known varieties of domesticated apples. We regularly eat about five.

The seemingly broad range of food that's readily available to us—which industrial food companies highlight with great pride—has been restricted to a short list of staple items. Most of them are poured into animal feed or processed food. So many aspects of today's food system provoke appropriate outrage. But this funneling of potentially endless food choices into the narrowest of channels, for the worst possible reasons, should top the list.

The figures backing up this point are alarming. No less than 75 percent of the world's food derives from five animals and twelve plants. Nearly 60 percent of all human-consumed plant calories derive from three plants—rice, corn, and wheat. *There are an estimated 50,000 edible plants in existence.* There are also thousands of edible, minimally non-sentient animals populating the lower depths of the food web. Still, the average American gets almost all of his meat—about 220 lbs. a year on average —from cows, pigs, and chickens.[2] It's as if a voracious reader walked into the New York Public Library every day and, every time, read the same book. As television chef Gordon Ramsey is prone to telling his anxious amateur chefs who oversear the tuna or undercook the flan: *What a shame.*

Appreciate this disparity between what exists and what could exist

---

2. http://www.npr.org/sections/thesalt/2012/06/27/155527365/visualizing-a-nation-of-meat-eaters

in terms of our diet and the ambition of this book begins to come into focus: It is our failure to access this vast cornucopia of taste, texture, and nutrition—our failure to eat promiscuously from what could be rather than what is—that's at the root of our dysfunctional food system.

As we imagine what a future food system might look like, as we accept the creative challenge of starting from scratch, it's imperative that we also consider ideas that support a vast range of low-impact plant and animal foods, produced and acquired in the wisest, most sustainable ways, as regular sources of nutrition. This move toward diversity requires us to reconsider the very act of eating. The goal of this book is, in a way, to help facilitate that vision.

Why do we eat what we eat? Why do we eat as much as we eat? Why do we eat where we eat? Why do we find some food gross and other food "clean?" Why do we accept some foods as normal but reject others? I don't necessarily answer these questions in what lies ahead (although I touch on all of them). Nothing that follows is gospel. Eating promiscuously may not be the only way to escape 12,000 years of agricultural confinement and oppression. But I think it's an important way to begin this kind of thought experiment. It bears on all of us. Even the most privileged eaters—even the most knowledgeable and educated among us—don't come remotely close to eating as well as we might be eating. Our eating habits are so engrained in endless unexamined conventions that we sometimes don't even understand them to be habits that can be changed.

To a large extent, we are victims. We are victims of our own narrow-minded success, a success that confines our imagination and perpetuates a system that's ruinous to our health and the planet itself. The whole foundational idea of what it means for a modern human to eat food has been severely compromised by a history of decisions that we have, through no necessary fault of our own, inherited. Our incredibly productive efficiency has resulted in innumerable conveniences. But when it comes to food its promise to make life easier has worked out all too well. Today's food system, with its underlying reality of culinary monotony existing beneath the guise of endless choice, represents the unintended outcome of a million small decisions and good intentions. But the sum total has added up to a disaster. We shouldn't accept it.

It's taken me a while to reach this conclusion. Earlier, I was more hopeful. I thought humans might achieve meaningful reform by tampering with the system within the boundaries of global agriculture. What was needed, I argued in my previous book *Just Food*, was balance—a judicious blend of various agricultural approaches, perhaps a merging of organic and conventional production, dramatically reduced meat consumption, the careful use of genetic modification, and the intelligent application of additional agricultural technologies to achieve the highest yields on the least amount of land.

But this plan was shortsighted. What I failed to realize was that the system I was promoting was quite hopelessly beyond help. The measures I proposed, I later realized, did almost nothing to promote the kind of diversity the food system needs. I was blinded by the very walls I wanted to expand, unaware of how they contained my thinking, channeled me into a groove of thought that locked down too many assumptions about agricultural change as sacred truth.

Later, in *The Modern Savage*, I addressed a more precise concern: meat. This time I argued in a more extreme direction, suggesting that the only solution to this dilemma was veganism, or at least something as close to a plant-based diet as we could get. In the context of today's dietary options, veganism certainly has considerable merit. Notably, it does more than any other diet to reduce the ecological problems that plague industrial agriculture. It's also, I believe, a highly effective way to lessen the suffering of animals we know to be fully sentient. This is a concern that, as we'll repeatedly see in the pages ahead, is essential to any future food system that claims to be just.

Again, though, I got it wrong. It was short sighted to think that there was some sort of magic answer to be found in the pursuit of a strictly plant-based diet. I never fully appreciated how veganism failed to think systematically beyond the boundaries of traditional agriculture, how it failed to promote the radical kind of culinary diversity that could save our health and the health of the planet. The more I attended "veg conferences" across the country, the more I edged toward this conclusion. Encountering vegans who were as likely to be unhealthy as healthy, in addition to the dogged promotion of salty and highly processed meat substitutes, I realized yet again how the system that contained veganism was still calling the shots. It struck me as a diet trying to turn the battleship by pushing on the boat from the inside.

None of this is to suggest that there aren't real virtues to be found in some popular alternative diets. Veganism—in addition to the organic and paleo options—reflects a much needed effort to achieve some measure of dietary discipline. Any effort to impose principles upon an otherwise unfettered food culture, and to draw a rough road map through an altogether confusing and often deceptive culinary landscape, should be considered progress. These efforts, as far as they go, can be admired for their assertive approach to a food system that's otherwise happy to make decisions for us, turning us into passive consumers. But, once again, they are, on balance, nowhere near enough to undo the problem and by helping us to reimagine a genuine solution.

The underlying issue with these dietary strategies is that they seek solutions with existing tools that are now at our disposal instead of using tools of our own creation. They stick with what is rather than asking what could be. They are not, in and of themselves, effective at promoting a fundamentally new kind of dietary thought, a basic rethinking of what it means to produce food, to consume food, and to foster a future food culture that's global in scope but looks nothing like what came before it.

Proof lies in how the currently popular alternatives diets—let's stick with vegan, paleo, and organic—have thus far fared. They have generally failed to support the very standards they espouse. They have failed not because they are terrible ideas. They aren't. But they have failed for the simple reason that, in the framework of today's food culture, they are necessarily undermined. Like a flame denied oxygen, they suffocate into nothingness. I present the following overview of failure not to criticize or condemn those who stick to these programs. Rather, I want to highlight the limitations of seeking reform within the current paradigm, one that quashes even the most concerted and thoughtful efforts to seek reform from within.

Paleo dieters want to eat how humans ate prior to the transition to agriculture. They limit themselves to meat, fruits, nuts, and root vegetables while avoiding refined carbs, potatoes, grain, and most legumes. Paleos appear to do well on this selection of food—at least in terms of weight loss (the medical benefits are not yet fully known). But the big drawback is that the food available today comes almost entirely from domesticated sources. The meat and plants paleo dieters eat are, in terms of nutritional profiles, light years away from their wild forbears. It's a difference of kind more than a difference of degree; it undercuts the inherent justification of the diet. In an age of prefabricated food, it's hard to eat like a caveman.

Vegans, for their part, seek to avoid all animal products. Most do so to reduce unnecessary animal suffering. But this endeavor fails to account for the billions of animals (squirrels, field mice, rabbits, etc.) killed to produce the plants and plant-based foods that vegans exclusively eat. Growing plants, in fact, almost surely kills more animals that would be killed if we simply replaced most of our plant-based calories with the flesh of large animals raised on grass. This is a tough reality for the vegan to confront. But it definitely effects the diet's founding justification. The bottom line here is that agriculture, whether plant or animal based, kills animals. Lots of them.

Supporters of organic agriculture also run into problems. They claim that their food choices—mostly produced without synthetic chemical inputs—are healthier for their bodies and the environment. But evidence on both claims is sketchy at best. Organic agriculture generally suffers lower yields. It does so while using pesticides that, although "all-natural," are sometimes more dangerous than chemical ones. It is not, according to several meta-studies, necessarily healthier than their conventional counterparts. Just because something is "natural" does not make it better.

In the end, each diet is effectively stymied by the food system that contains them.

The implication here should be clear: If we're going to look beyond what's currently been placed under our noses—what we have, through no fault of our own, inherited from previous generations—we must think beyond popular dietary alternatives. We have to consider a starkly different kind of food system, one that's more diversified, geared towards nurturing culinary promiscuity, and, in turn, one which is primed for optimal health, ecological justice, and complete transparency and accessibility. We need to work harder to know the unknowns. Obviously, this is not an easy task.

My "starting over" thought experiment does not require tossing overboard *everything* that came before. I'm all for preserving the productive elements within each of the aforementioned diets. Most notably, in so far as each diet encourages a move away from the corn-soy-animal agriculture (and refined sugar) complex, the more it should be included in our vision. But as we'll see in the pages ahead, a truly diverse and altered food system will demand more than these diets can offer. It will require going far beyond the assumptions that inform these alternative ways of eating. It will mean conceptualizing the plant and animal world in a much broader way, transcending the organic/conventional distinction, and avoiding the starchy staple crops that bring us so many processed carbs and sugars. None of these diets accomplishes these goals on their own terms. They don't even do so together. If only due to the food system that contains them, these diets are, in the end, fads that inform our identity better than they reform the food system.

The best diet is no diet at all. This best diet is one we don't have to think about. We should allow ourselves to envision a food system that doesn't require us to negotiate it as if it were a minefield. We should not be expected to be as discerning as we currently have to be. We should not have to fight so diligently against food to be healthy.

To that end, the elimination of conventional farm animals from modern agriculture is the single most important prerequisite for accomplishing these goals. Imagining a new food system requires highlighting and understanding the ecological and welfare implications of factory-farmed animals. Fortunately, critics of industrial agriculture have been brilliant in accomplishing this goal. If any one feature has characterized the food writing of the last twenty years, it is the dismantling of the logic behind industrial animal agriculture.

Where the critics fall short, though, is in what they almost always do next: suggesting that returning all those animals to pasture, and raising them under natural conditions, will somehow solve the problem of factory farming. This more humane arrangement might work in certain local contexts, and under certain precise conditions. But pasture-based animal agriculture is neither scalable nor supportive of future culinary diversity. It does very little to shunt resources away from the beef, chicken, and pork grown in modern factories to serve a food system that allows us to be promiscuous in our dietary choices.

Whether on pasture or confined into factories, today's farm animals currently consume the majority of the global food system's limited natural resources. Plus, with their higher order cognition and their clear sense of self, they account for the most extensive suffering within agriculture (chickens bear the brunt of this burden). Cruel as it sounds, these animals do not belong on pasture for the basic reason that they do not belong *anywhere*. They are, as is the case with all the food we eat, beings of our own creation, beings whose presence alone, whether confined or free-ranged, makes it virtually impossible for us to tap into a hidden world of plant and animal diversity.

The kind of animal agriculture that's focused on large land-based animals who are sentient, social, and, in the case of pigs, probably able to outwit your five-year old honor student, cannot be sustained. The animals we now eat—the ones in the stores and on the menus—can really have only one permanent destination: gradual extinction.

♡◯◔

The numbers help illuminate why. In the United States alone, the majority of arable land and water goes to producing over 10 billion animals—
again, mostly chickens—for human consumption. Putting animals on
pasture would only worsen the pressure on land and water. The tyr-
anny of corn and soy on the American landscape, which is a necessary
counterpart to commercial animal production, reflects our irrational
dedication to these resource-intensive creatures. Because of corn and
soy, and because land animals are so resource intensive, animal agriculture is one of the world's leading causes of ecological destruction. It's
a major source of greenhouse gas emissions (about 14 percent, larger
than transportation), consumes 75 percent of the water in drought-
prone regions such as the American West, and accounts (again through
corn and soy-based feed) for the majority of nitrogen fertilizer runoff,
which leads to dead zones in places such as the Gulf of Mexico. It's
the primary cause of biodiversity loss due to increasingly rapid rates
of deforestation.

In consuming these resources—air, water, land, biodiversity—animal agriculture does more than diminish our health and that of the environment. It also burdens us with attendant opportunity costs. Namely, it
prevents us from pursuing more creative and productive ways of allocat-
ing those resources to foster a more diverse diet. Every agricultural decision we make hides agricultural decisions we didn't make. The inputs
that go towards fattening a cow are inputs that didn't go towards building a vertical vegetable farm. This kind of zero-sum analysis has largely
been absent in discussions of food and agricultural reform.

So when people talk about agriculture being such a horrific disaster,
it is precisely this tragic misallocation of natural resources to corn, soy,
and animals to which they refer. And while the idea of replacing corn
and soy with grass and other forage is seductive, it's a decision that still
requires using considerable resources to grow alfalfa hay (which all grass
fed cows eat), to graze the animals on extensive plots of land that could
be otherwise employed, and to quench their thirst (a dairy cow needs
twenty gallons of water a day)[3] with water that could be conserved or put

---

3. http://extension.oregonstate.edu/douglas/sites/default/files/documents/lf/WATERLF0503.pdf

to better use. It's a decision that consumes those resources to promote the monocultural production of a few kinds of meat rather than using those resources to achieve a more diverse system that encourages us to eat more thoughtfully from a vast spectrum of healthier choices.

Animal agriculture kills our agricultural dreams. It prevents us from accessing a world of foods and flavors that require the same resources currently invested in chicken, pork, and beef. The first step we need to take before envisioning a new way to eat is to identify animal agriculture as the primary obstacle to achieving a reformed food system. Given that Americans eat 220 pounds of this kind of meat per person per year, this will require a big erasure. When I mention the idea of sending conventional land animals into existential oblivion, my friends react as if I suggested we go out and slaughter infants. After choking on their bacon cheeseburgers, they bristle with righteous indignation. I'm going to *deny* them the rapture of Texas barbeque!?

Well, yes. But, as I then tell them, consider the other side of the equation. Look at what your barbecue has done to my culinary options. Acknowledge what we are missing out on because of our cultural addiction to a few choice cuts of meat. Again, the opportunity costs. Barbecue and other resource intensive foods are preventing our access to thousands of foods and flavors and nutrient profiles for which the resources are otherwise occupied. That's thousands of tastes and textures for the singular indulgence of a plate of barbeque?

Seems a little unfair to me. I'd rather give up the BBQ and have access to those other foods and flavors. So would my health. So would the environment. And, for what it's worth, so would the animals.

Accessing a new world of food and flavor requires largely eliminating the old world of food and flavor. The idea that the food system we have created, based on a somewhat bizarre arrangement known as agriculture, is something we have done well, gotten right, and served us well, is naïve. It blinds us to the evolutionary fact that modern humans, although we have inherited agriculture from our recent ancestors, are even more so the trustees of millions of years of food choices made by very distant predecessors who, before the turn to agriculture, knew a lot more about healthy eating than we do today.

But how could we access the wisdom these ancestors, known as they are only through the bounty of their bones? One way might be to explore the diet of a close non-human relative. When my thoughts about expanding our palates by radically diversifying the food system were starting to percolate, I shared them with John Mackey, the founder and co-CEO of Whole Foods. John listened and, as he has a way of doing, immediately took my thoughts, jumped the species barrier, and packaged them into a pithy catchphrase. "You're describing the Bonobo diet," he said. "Bonobos eat that way." *That's good,* I thought.

A bonobo is in many ways an ideal guide for how we might shift the way we think about food. It eats largely but not exclusively plants; the plants the bonobo eats are diverse and devoid of starchy staple crops; bonobos complement these plants with an impressive range of lower-order animal foods, namely insects and grubs, which they eat in small amounts throughout the day; some of the bonobos' relatives (the macaque) eat shellfish; and bonobos are radically flexible in what they will consume, keeping their palates open to all kinds of venture and experimentation. (Bonobos also have sex five times a day. But I digress).

This book is not going to make the case that humans ought to eat (or behave) exactly like chimps. In fact, this book will prescribe no formal diet whatsoever. But its goals are such that the bonobo offers the guidance of a sort of spirit animal, both embodying and symbolizing the range and openness that humans might bring to the food system. In general, this book will explore how we can think about the future human diet in terms that, although largely unfamiliar, have deep resonance in a lost history of diversity that, today, the bonobos instinctively exploit. It will, in this regard, attempt to imagine a food system that mostly rejects the current food production paradigm, embraces the diverse consumption of underexploited (or unexploited) plants and animals, and, in a move that takes us beyond the bonobos, envisions a food future that's as humane, sustainable, and as globally accessible as we can make it (rather than available only to elite foodies, who, as will become clear, are a special kind of thorn in my side).

In this sense, consider what follows not as a precise guide to food choice, food policy, personal diet, or specific agricultural reform strategies. Rather, consider it a bonobo-inspired attempt to promote a new way to think about eating. See it as a spur to our collective imagination about what the human diet could be—an attempt to foster a mentality that accepts real change, whatever form it takes, and allows that change to grow into forms now unknown.

This book explores the idea of a future food system by profiling various people who, in various ways, are already innovating under the assumption that, when it comes to eating, we must remove ourselves from what came before. They are outliers who are, by their various quests, already tuned in to the bonobo agenda. They are pursuing peripheral culinary goals informed by principles that lead us further astray from conventional thinking and ever closer to the ideal of starting over. Collectively they combine the spirit of pre-agrarian foodways with contemporary technology. They've already nurtured an intuitive understanding of promiscuous eating, approached achieving it in a variety of fascinating ways, and developed principles about food that, if popularized, have the potential to revolutionize how we think about the human diet. They are uncomfortable with what is. They look to what could be.

Their exceptional nature is critical to what follows. In so many areas of life, it's the outcast, the freak, the loner on the periphery—often the distant periphery—who ends up having the best idea. Although largely overlooked, the figures I profile are way ahead of the status quo when it comes to nurturing ambitions that are, in various ways, bonobo-like. They are unbound by convention, inspired by an inner instinct, and beholden to no interests other than the pull of their own idiosyncratic vision. However unwittingly, and for whatever reason, these people permit themselves to think differently. Their rules are not ordinary, and they are exactly the kind of rules that could lead us toward a fundamentally better way to eat.

Steve Jobs put it better: "Here's to the crazy ones, the misfits, the rebels, the troublemakers, the round pegs in the square holes... the ones who see things differently — they're not fond of rules... You can quote them, disagree with them, glorify or vilify them, but the only thing you can't do is ignore them because they change things... they push the human race forward, and while some may see them as the crazy ones, we see genius, because the ones who are crazy enough to think that they can change the world, are the ones who do."

Amen.

In presenting these figures, I'm in no way suggesting that, as concerned consumers, we need to emulate them (no more than we need to emulate bonobo chimps). I'm not saying that, to usher in a radically new food system based on a different set of premises about what it means to eat, we need to go dumpster diving, or hunter-gathering, or undertake a comprehensive lifestyle transition, or tinker with plant DNA, or harvest seaweed or grow insects, or become a connoisseur of road kill, a weekend boar hunter, or an oyster farmer. We'll see all of these ambitions manifested in the pages ahead. But I'm not saying you should necessarily go out and do them.

Given how little progress we have made in reforming the food system, even after decades of identifying it as broken, my intention is more reflective than instructive. As we investigate unconventional approaches to acquiring food, as we look to the periphery for principles that might one day inform the center, I'm hopeful we can discover ideas that will begin to illuminate the opening question: *what if we could start over?* I've embraced the outliers not only for what they are doing. But for how their efforts inform a new culinary imagination, a post-agricultural mode of thought that exceeds anything that ever came before us, placing most of the agricultural past in the dustbin.

The enlightenment political philosopher and, in his own way, revolutionary thinker, Edmund Burke argued that every generation held moral duties not only to itself but to future generations. When it comes to agriculture, 12,000 years' worth of ancestral attempts to grow food has badly served that responsibility. Generation upon generation has left us with food that we have every right to wish we never inherited. Burke's philosophical counterpart, Thomas Jefferson, took a different stance on generational responsibility, arguing that we should, with each generational turn, cut all ties with those who preceded us. "The earth," he wrote to James Madison, "belongs in usufruct to the living." The time has come to borrow from Jefferson so we can, as proper custodians of food's future, honor Burke.

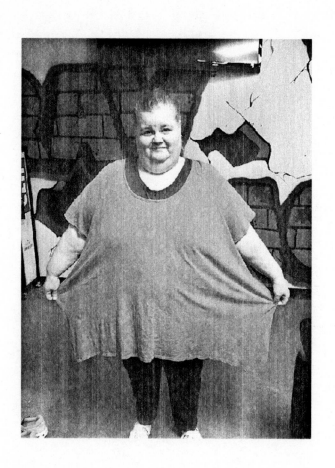

# CHAPTER ONE

# The Paradox of Abundance

*"For man, unlike any other thing organic or inorganic in the universe, grows beyond his work, walks up the stairs of his concepts, emerges ahead of his accomplishments."*
—JOHN STEINBECK, *The Grapes of Wrath*

There's an insect that's dreaded by vegetable farmers called the squash borer. Squash borers lay their eggs deep inside the fibrous stem of a plant and, the moment the larvae hatch, they begin tunneling their way out, consuming what's directly in front of them. They don't nibble. They devour with evolutionary urgency. For the farmer, this obnoxious (if brilliant) example of parasitic adaptation results in succulent gourds being reduced to a pile of mush. For the insects, it means the necessary fuel to sustain them during their sex-fueled month on earth. One side wins; the other loses. Hello, nature.

This is an apt analogy for consumers trying to negotiate today's warmed over buffet of commercial food choices. Only in this case the winners and losers are reversed. The average American who eats what the industrial food system has placed before him—be it at the school cafeteria, restaurants, or the grocery store—will most likely become overweight, perhaps obese, and possibly sick as a direct result of that decision. The food companies that mix and remix variations of starch, salt, sugar, and fat into endless and irresistible concoctions, not to mention the pharmaceutical companies that manufacture the drugs to treat the resulting illnesses, are the ones having the party.

The situation has a fish-in-water quality to it. It's easy to never notice the abundance in which we swim. Still, we're currently experiencing a phenomenon that humans have never before experienced: A food system that we must actively fight against, with every ounce of discipline and education we have, in order to stay even moderately healthy. Not to overstate the case, but we're trapped and surrounded by an awful selection of food that has hijacked our taste buds, imprisoned our bodies, and compromised our abilities to make common sense choices about what we eat. The lifelines by which to escape are few. Before exploring how we might save escape this situation, we first need to ask: How did we even get here in the first place?

## A BRIEF HISTORY OF OBESITY

There are reasons for our increasingly supersized condition. In *The Story of the Human Body*, Daniel Lieberman, a Harvard evolutionary biologist, helps explain the dilemma in which we now find ourselves. The human body we inhabit today essentially evolved to be active. More than any other physical demand, humans required energy to fulfill the need to move—and move a lot—and the body we inherited reflects that ongoing demand. Pre-agrarian patterns of hunting, gathering, and scavenging meant covering about 9.3 miles a day. That's about 20,000 steps on your fitbit.

Factor in all the climbing, bending, lifting, and stretching required for common food acquisition (and other activities) and the overall physical demands become even more extensive. Our organs, our limbs, our gluteus muscles, even the heels that keep us upright—were honed by a long stretch of evolution to foster excessive mobility geared for food production and processing, thereby allowing the slow burn of constant physical endurance to sustain us through long days on the savannah. We may or may not have been born to run. But we were definitely born to use our bodies for constant physical work.

The impressive array of foods humans acquired and ate before agriculture—roots, nuts, fruits, vegetables, game, seaweed, shellfish, fish, and so on—evolved to complement our considerable level of energy expenditure. What ensued over time was a fine equipoise between energy intake and physical activity. It was a balance that, generally speaking, served us well. It's commonly noted that pre-agrarian human bodies were taller than modern humans, held more erectly, and endowed with denser bones. Nothing here should be romanticized. A pre-agrarian scavenging life was in many ways a merciless existence that none of us should really want to revisit. Famine was always a good possibility. There were no vaccines or antibiotics to prevent diseases from killing us. The hunter could be mauled by a lion or toppled from a dugout canoe and swallowed by the sea. I'll take cold beer and advanced medicine over most of what these cave dwellers had to deal with.

But the scavenger was also likely not going to die from a "lifestyle disease." He ate foods that were in tune with his body in the way that today, I imagine, only elite athletes can perhaps approximate. There were, according to one researcher's investigation into the question, "few if any"[4] obese people. Additional weight was simply incommensurate with the patterns of human life, strenuous and stunted though that life might have been.

Then came farming. As humans transitioned to early forms of agriculture, the impressive physical rigors of working the land, in addition to the fact that everyone farmed with their own backs bent to the hoe, generally kept our inherited hunter-gatherer bodies in fine form. Not only were humans taller than we are now, but the rigor of agrarian labor staved off the first rise of obesity until about the 5th century BC. It was then that early signs of gluttony (of a Falstaffian sort) started to fatten the Greek populace's loafing-prone, slave-holding elite. Athenian physician Hippocraties was attuned to this subtle trend, observing the not-so-subtle outcome that overweight people did something earlier more often than thin people besides eat: they died.[5]

---

4. http://www.slate.com/articles/news_and_politics/explainer/2009/05/old_and_fat.html
5. http://www.ncbi.nlm.nih.gov/pubmed/2276853; http://www.internationaljournalofcardiology.com/article/S0167-5273(05)01231-3/abstract

For a couple thousand years this heft—perhaps because it was linked with wealth—conferred social benefits. Extra girth became a status symbol for wealthier men while the curvy "Rubenesque" formation assumed the voluptuous ideal for leisured women. But by the eighteenth-century, as agricultural surpluses became increasingly available to the wealthier classes, especially in modernizing places such as early America and Europe, (where global trade in food was increasing), this extra weight trickled down to the masses. It was on the lower rungs of the socioeconomic ladder, as the hips and bellies of the hoi-polloi swelled, that obesity was downgraded from a status marker to a medical condition, if not sometimes a stigma. As early as 1863 there were already diet books on the market. While relatively few people were officially obese, the problem was, nonetheless, officially that—a problem.

The onset of late-19th- and early 20th-century industrialization democratized the problem of being overweight. It transformed obesity from a rare but noteworthy condition into something so common that, today, it afflicts nearly 40 percent of the American population. Whereas an obese person was once considered a rarity, a person you might secretly stare at, today he no longer warrants a second look. "More die in the United States of too much food than of too little," the economist John Kenneth Galbraith could aptly observe by the middle of the 20th century. Matters have only worsened since the famous economist's observation.

How did this transition happen in such a brief span of time? As Lieberman explains, industrialization plucked our active bodies from the field and locked them into an increasingly sedentary routine (a trend that digital life has only worsened). Humans living in an industrial society experienced enormous material benefits, as have humans living in a digital society. But, in terms of holistic bodily health, we've suffered.

Humans went from burning around 5000 calories a day (as working farmers) to about 2000 as sedentary office and industrial workers.6 Never in the whole history of work had such a dramatic shift in kinetic behavior occurred so abruptly. Industrial agriculture, meanwhile, stocked the shelves around our lethargic selves with subsidized and calorically dense

6. http://www.livestrong.com/article/278257-how-many-calories-does-the-body-naturally-burn-per-day/; http://calorielab.com/burned/?mo=se&gr=11&ti=Occupation&wt=150&un=lb&kg=68

food, placing all of it within arms reach, keeping it ultra cheap, and making the least healthy food the most tempting to eat. For the prospects of rapid weight gain, this was the perfect storm.

The food, moreover, is addictive. More than anything else that humans have ever consumed, industrially processed food presents a burst of taste and "mouthfeel" that's alarmingly consistent and irresistible. It captivates us with scientifically tested combinations of sweet, salty, and savory sensations, the alchemistic outcome of a deep but insidious brand of research that's designed to do nothing more than push the product onto the defenseless palates of unsuspecting consumers. A small sign on the ice cream case at a neighborhood ice cream shop reads, "Feel the butterfat on the roof of your mouth." It is with these words that industrial foods seduced us into passivity.

Mark Shatzker, author of *The Dorito Effect,* has explored this phenomenon in some depth. He writes, "Flavor factories churn out chemical desire. We spray, squirt, and inject hundreds of millions of pounds of those chemicals on food every year, and then we find ourselves surprised and alarmed that people keep eating." For most of us it is hard—and for some seemingly impossible—to resist the routine offerings of the industrial food system. Try eating just one salty, freshly fried tortilla chip. Good luck. The chemists who engineer how we will experience a food's intensity and texture are smarter and less scrupulous than our weak and suggestible palates. Food has inherently addictive qualities. The experience of eating today thus leaves us deeply satisfied in the moment but, in the long run, prone to lifestyle diseases that follow from that alluring promise of orgasmic pleasure.

As an empirical matter, our bodies have responded pretty much as you'd expect. Measures of Body Mass Index (BMI) between 1882 and 1986 capture the extent of the change. Among eighteen-year-old men, BMIs rose modestly, from 19.9 to 20.1 by the turn of the 20th century. Between 1909 and 1920, it rose a bit higher, from 20.1 to 22.3, where it held steady until the 1950s. But then, just as the postwar economy kicked into high gear, and just as the food system reached new levels of industrialization (as a result of better farming through chemistry), the average personal BMI skyrocketed. Between 1950 and 1986, it went from 22.4 to 24.2. All told, over a hundred years, the average eighteen-year old became twenty-nine pounds heavier.

Today, it is even larger, with an average BMI around 24.5. It's no wonder we've become as susceptible as we've ever been to heart disease, diabetes, strokes, and hypertension.[7] As Michael Pollan has written, with an appropriate tone of alarm, obesity "is arguably the most pressing public health problem we face."[8]

## ASSIGNING BLAME

Explaining how obesity came about is less challenging than explaining why. Is it that modern and digitized humans have abandoned all self-control? That we've become weak willed and gluttonous? I wish the case were so simple. But it's not.

It is easy, and it is tempting, and it even feels kind of good, to lay the blame for obesity squarely on the obese. In a culture that values (rhetorically at least) individualism and personal accountability, not to mention an abundance of accurate nutritional information (more and more of it required by legislation), it seems perfectly reasonable to hold people ultimately responsible for the food they consume and the physical consequences—not to mention the health care costs—that predictably follow.

Medical doctors lean in this direction all the time. They remind their patients, over and over again, with mounting frustration, that obesity is strictly a physical problem. It comes down to calories consumed versus calories burned. Of course, as a matter of cold logic, this assessment is true. But the implications around thinking this way are such that a person becomes overweight because a) he can't count, b) has no self-control, c) doesn't care; and d) all of the above.

I'm not prepared to circle any of these answers. I understand the appeal of blaming the vicitm. Still, I'm not ready to do it. For one, I don't think it's especially compassionate. But more so, there are other less empirical factors that contribute to obesity, and while one of those

7. http://www.voxeu.org/article/100-years-us-obesity
8. The Omnivore's Dilemma.

factors is indeed sometimes a basic failure of will, or chronic lack of discipline, or even a complete indifference to one's bodily integrity, I still believe that, on the whole, the obese among us have succumbed to forces largely beyond their control and hard to identify. Generally speaking, the obese aren't weak willed or devoid of ability to live measured lives. They don't want to be obese. They're trapped.

They are victims. They're victims of a food system that demeans their health and wellbeing at every turn. They're victims of an agricultural inheritance that insults them with calorically dense junk food. They're victims of a culture that requires us to spend too much time staring at screens, sitting at desks, and driving in cars. They're victims of municipal planning and suburban sprawl that turns walking and biking into high-adventure hazards (seriously: try walking ten miles anywhere in a city such as Atlanta or Houston or Denver and you'll appreciate this claim; hell, just try walking ten miles anywhere). They're victims, far too often, of widespread economic injustice, the kind that leads to a sense of scarcity so psychologically devastating that it drives the least prosperous among us to consume foods that are cheap, dense, and awful for our health (more on this in a moment). They are also victims, as we will see, of personal traumas that lead many people to eat as the only form of relief from their suffering.

This trap I'm describing isn't all encompassing. People avoid it all the time—usually wealthier people, those with access to the best schools, mental health care, leisure time, and supportive social and familial networks. Many of us have had the excellent good fortune—and perhaps the genes—to lead lives with healthy, weight-appropriate bodies. We've enjoyed a health-conscious upbringing, a sound nutritional education, economic prosperity, an advanced degree, an urban life replete with sidewalks and bike lanes, and perhaps an early-developed habit of high fiber and rigorous exercise. These attributes often allow us to intelligently negotiate the food system.

There's also sociology to consider. The lucky few surround each other. We discuss health-related issues. We're aware that grocery stores and restaurant menus are full of pitfalls. We know about "added fat" and "empty calories." We show restraint when it comes to processed foods. When we do indulge in unhealthy food (usually high-end unhealthy food), we do so knowing that the indulgence must be a rarity, a treat. More often than not, we affirm each other's smart health choices; we socialize each other through our words, ideas, and habits. Our ability to manage a healthy lifestyle in a generally toxic food environment becomes, in this respect, inbred. And so we escape. Good for us. We're lucky to have this ability.

But even the lucky few are vulnerable. Their situation is not as stable as we might assume. Not everyone is as healthy as they could be, or even thinks themselves to be. Lack of obesity hardly connotes the presence of optimal physical health. Eating fruits and vegetables, avoiding processed foods, and exercising daily, under current conditions, may not be enough to avoid the lifestyle diseases that plague us at such high rates. We might work diligently to stay fit and trim but, even so, the most nutritionally educated (and otherwise educated) among us must still struggle to maintain dietary discipline.

In the United States obesity might be at 35 percent. But potassium deficiency is at 90 percent; 80 percent of us are vitamin E deficient, 70 percent are calcium deficient, and half of us are deficient in vitamin A, C, D, and magnesium.[9] "Hidden hunger," this condition is sometimes called. Even eating well within the pre-existing options by no means guarantees we'll avoid suffering health problems as a result of our food choices. Even the commonly assumed healthy diet, the one eaten by the high-end shoppers at boutique grocery stores and farmers' markets, may not be all we think it to be.

There's also the possibility of the lucky few gradually slipping toward weight gain and poor health. A number of factors can instigate this decline. Anecdotally, I've seen it happen a lot, especially in recent years, as my cohort of peers enters their forties. Several friends and family members who are supremely health conscious, friends who shop on the peripheries of grocery stores and order judiciously at restaurants,

9. https://www.caltonnutrition.com/micronutrient-deficiency-pandemic/; http://www.dsm.com/campaigns/talkingnutrition/en_US/talkingnutrition-dsm-com/2015/03/nutrient_deficiencies_among_US_adolescents.html

and exercise regularly, still manage to put on weight. They have returned from annual physicals, in some cases, baffled by news that they're somehow "pre-diabetic." This is not the natural result of aging. It's the food system. It's the choice available under the guise of abundance. It's what surrounds us.

When members of an intense running group to which I belong must stop running for a relatively short period of time (say a couple of months), usually due to an injury, they'll quickly gain an observable amount of weight in the interim if they do not do some cross training. When a friend's mother recently became seriously ill, the time he put into caring for his mom derailed him from his normally healthy diet and gym routine. He gained an alarming amount of weight in a matter of months. Another friend, an ultra-marathoner in his fifties with a PhD has put on weight when he had to do an excessive amount of travelling for work.

I realize these anecdotes might seem either meaningless or the perfectly logical outcome of a quick shift to inactivity. But at the same time, something doesn't seem right. As I interpret these admittedly anecdotal cases, they strike me as sobering testimonies to the food environment in which we're trapped. It's what happens when we stay still, or even only get a little less active, and eat—even intelligently—from the food trough that's currently placed under our nose by companies promising to enrich our lives with an abundance of food.

The only people I know who consistently maintain excellent fitness levels, marked by healthy body weight, are men and women (many of them well into their seventies) who follow a fanatically structured diet and exercise routine, often to such an extreme that people think they're clinically obsessed. In fact they are not clinically obsessed. They've just been able to discover an elusive sweet spot, striking a balance among kinetic movement, dietary diversity, and the right amount of calories consumed in a culinary milieu that they've managed to figure out. They have threaded a needle, negotiating industrial food and post-industrial sedentariness to live more or less as their bodies evolved for them to live, at ease in their optimal physical selves.

♡○○

So, to reiterate: As it currently stands, the options in front of us too often and too easily culminate in obesity, or at least excessive weight gain, for the majority of the U.S. population. Even those who work diligently to fight against such a common fate succumb to it. It's a frustrating and unfair situation. Thirty-six percent of us are obese; two-thirds carry more weight than they should; 80 percent fail to eat the recommended daily allowance of fruits and vegetables. And, the kicker: we're in denial.

According to a recent study, 75 percent of us believe that we're eating a perfectly adequate diet—that we're healthy. What we fail to realize (understandably) is that we make this assessment in the face of what is in front of us rather than what could be. It's a situation that you can be sure Big Pharma is happy to treat with increasingly expensive drugs and other medical therapies. But, as we are about to see, it's a situation that can, with herculean effort, be escaped.

It's perfectly possible to become liberated from the fat trap. Not easy, not without help, not without big changes, but possible. To understand the radical extremes we must go to in order to rescue our bodies from a deranged food system (complemented by a sedentary culture), I followed the three-month journey of a family from Austin, Texas, three individuals who became stuck in the food system much in the way I've described above. Recognizing that they were on a fast track to an early death, they made a collective decision to opt out of the food system as they knew it.

## MEET THE REEDS

The Reed family—Becca (51), James (57), and their son Drew (26)—lives in Austin, Texas. The first thing to say about their collective decision to become healthy within the current food paradigm is that it's hard to fathom. They were sick. There were few precedents for what they are doing. They were determined to change.

Their raw will, leavened with basic human decency, turned my journalistic objectivity into advocacy. I wanted to be a stenographer to their success as they emerged (as the opening Steinbeck quotes alludes) ahead of their accomplishments. I met or spoke with them several times a week for many months to cover their experience on the road to wellness. Their openness was almost disarming. "Ask us anything," Becca said after a month. "We'll give an answer."

They did. I'm opening this book with their story because it offers a baseline. Specifically, it demonstrates something critical about our current food system, as well as the sedentary lifestyle it encourages. Getting trapped is not only easy to do, but it's a burden so oppressive that, for many of us, the only way out it is to become an entirely different kind of person—to reshape our sense of self. Becca Reed, during her first week of training, told me as much. She said that she and her family wanted "to become new people" as they undertook the campaign to save themselves. "We want to be *better* people," she added.

Their experience does much more than remind us how easy it is to become obese in today's food culture. Their effort to escape the standard American diet also sparks our imagination in a bolder way. It inspires questions that, in our obsession with diet, weight, and body image, we rarely consider asking: What if the food in front us, the food we habitually consume, didn't require us to think about it—to fight it—in order to have healthy bodies? What if we lived in a food culture so sane—so infused with products and values and standards of awareness that were commensurate with the bodies we were born into—rather than a system that makes us sick? What if we could, like the squash borer, wake up, eat, and thrive as a result of whatever we chose to put on our plates? What if the Reeds, as they escaped their condition, were able to find themselves amidst a food world that didn't require them to negotiate a food culture that wants to reclaim their health and happiness?

I had to witness the Reeds confront the food system to appreciate the importance of these questions. I had to watch them transform into new people to realize the inherent futility of trying to seek health in the current food system. If the Reeds have taught me anything about food—and, for that matter, about life—it is this: We have license to dream about a world you could once have never imagined existing.

♡○○

The Reeds have been obese for decades. But in the spring of 2016 they had hit rock bottom. Becca's diabetes (type II) was worsening. She was upping her insulin dosage daily. Her weight had ballooned to near 400 pounds, landing her in a wheelchair. She spent most of the day propped up in bed, watching television, and reading her Facebook page. Her son Drew spent his days bringing her food and medications.

Drew's recent gastric by-pass surgery, which he had back in December, left him 150 lbs. lighter. But he was still badly overweight and chronically lethargic. He was, as he'd long been, moody, always struggling to keep darkness at bay. This ongoing challenge, as it will do, inclined him to eat poorly, remain indoors, and spend his nights playing video games, sometimes until the sun came up.

James, also obese, had recently discovered that his already high blood pressure had further spiked to truly alarming levels (which meant another medication). He was coming home from his factory job (he mixes paint in a warehouse where there is no air conditioning) in increasingly foul moods. He would stomp into the house, brood, eat, watch TV, and get in bed, where his sleep Apnea would keep him snorting himself awake every ten minutes.

Altogether, the family was taking thirty-one medications.

Food was the main cause of their problems. The Reeds' diet consisted largely of industrial food's lowest hanging fruit: Taco Bell, Whataburger, Jack-N-the-Box, and, when they wanted to splurge, plate after plate of cheese-smothered Tex-Mex meals at Texican, a local chain. Their kitchen pantry reflected the middle aisles of the grocery store. Cookies, chips, crackers, and sugar-packed cereals—processed fare, all—were the norm. In other words: the American way of eating—to an extreme.

In a perverse kind of meal planning, the Reeds dedicated Sunday afternoons to mapping out which fast food restaurants they would frequent, and what they would order, for the upcoming week. More often than not James would pick up the food, usually at a nearby drive thru, bring it home, and the family would stare into a screen while eating off TV trays. Becca told me that, on some days, they would eat four different kinds of fast food, finishing the last meal within minutes of bedtime. As you might expect, the Reeds were doing more than super-sizing themselves. They were, alone together, slowly taking their own lives. James later told me he was certain he wouldn't live to see retirement.

One might blame the Reeds for killing themselves with this diet. As I suggested earlier, though, you might look at their situation another way—perhaps in a more charitable way—and alternatively conclude that the Reeds were in fact being killed. They were being victimized into poor health by a cheap, calorically dense, and easily accessible food supply that was enriching a handful of corporations and pharmaceutical companies as the expense of our bodies. I realize that this thesis may sound extreme  —and, honestly, until a few years ago, I wouldn't have bought it myself. But a recent body of research suggests that the victim thesis is more compelling than it might initially appear to be.

Start with one important topic at the center of our lives: financial resources. The Reeds, who pay a mortgage and can afford the basic amenities, nonetheless live close to the bone. It may not be a paycheck-to-paycheck situation, but they are by no means bursting with disposable income. Most would call them "middle class," but it's that precarious kind of middle class whereby Drew, when he developed a sharp pain in his stomach and wanted to see a doctor, couldn't afford to do so. At twenty-six, he's now off his dad's insurance plan, and has no formal job, caring as he does for his mother. So it's that kind of middle class.

In their book *Scarcity: Why Having Too Little Means So Much*, Sendhil Mullainathan and Eldar Shafir explore the impact of everyday scarcity on our basic choices. They explain how "scarcity captures the mind," how it's something that "has its own logic." They argue that it bears on all our decisions, including those related to food. It's not much of a leap, as they see it, to hypothesize that, if your entire material existence was teetering on the edge of loss—that is, if you were obsessed with scarcity because you were one minor car repair away from economic ruin—that you'd likely blow your limited food budget on junk food, naturally choosing a bag of cookies and fried chicken over some apples and kale. In a way, this choice makes sense. It's perfectly rational.

We're understandably wedded to the simple idea that, when it comes to eating, you reap what you sow. Calories go in, calories go out, and there's that gatekeeper—will power—in the middle. It's also understandable that we'd be impatient when so many people make poor choices in the face of accurate information telling them to do otherwise. Still, as Mullainathan and Shafir suggest, there are subtle sociological and psychological influences nudging our actions in less healthy directions. Scarcity is just one. But it is a powerful and, in many cases, hidden motivator that I think dramatically shapes the behavior of families such as the Reeds.

The Reeds don't want to be overweight. Their obesity is a condition that they despise. I'm thus even more inclined to accept the victim thesis. Either way you spin it, though, they were, in the early summer of 2016, in dire physical trouble.

♡O◌

On June 3, 2016, something happened that would significantly alter their lives. James and Becca read a story in a fitness magazine they had picked up in the lobby of the doctor's office. The article was a celebratory profile of a vegan-based gym in Austin owned and managed by a thirty-seven-year old trainer named Mike "Bonebreaker" Crockett. It wasn't veganism that drew James and Becca to the page; in fact, as Becca later told me, her "meat and potatoes upbringing" taught her that "vegans were weaklings." But it was Bonebreaker, the gym owner, who held their attention. Bald, with a golf ball-sized lump in the middle of his head, weighing in at over 400 pounds, sporting a braided ZZ-top beard, and adorned in tattoos that web around his arms, chest, and head, the man commands a double take.

The shock of Bonebreaker's appearance—and the fact that he didn't eat meat—was one thing. But there was something else that appealed to the Reeds: Bonebreaker isn't your typical gym rat—a lean and buff exemplar of bodily prowess. To the contrary, he's rough looking. He's from the sticks of poor, rural East Texas. Despite losing over 150 pounds over the last few years, he looks every bit the bar bouncer country boy he once was. This messier, slightly unhinged image appealed to the Reeds. Becca (and to a lesser extent James and Drew) is sensitive to being judged according to her appearance. A perfectly toned trainer would have been an immediate turn-off to her. (As I would later come to appreciate, this is not unusual; very fit people in general can be an unwitting source of discomfort for many obese people.)

Becca would almost certainly have ignored Bonebreaker if he looked like a gym owner. But, built like a tank and tattooed like a convict, he had soft blue eyes that looked just vulnerable enough to maybe have room in his heart for the Reeds' condition. James and Becca took the remarkable step of driving to the gym. They didn't necessarily see their initial visit in quite such therapeutic terms, but when they went to Bonebreaker's place, they were, in a way, reaching out for help.

Their intuition turned out to be right about at least one thing: Bonebreaker has a warm and generous heart. "I want to use my strength to help others," he later told me. He welcomed the Reeds, placing his twenty-five-inch biceps on their shoulders, and they all sat down to share their stories. As Becca talked (and Becca, we'd all learn, *talks*) about the family's descent into and struggle with obesity, Bonebreaker, who took careful notes, observed something in the Reeds that he knew all too well. He saw a form of addiction.

Five years earlier Bonebreaker had been faced with his own Manichean choice: death or sobriety. To aid his recovery, he also went vegetarian and, later, vegan. Kicking a fifteen-year habit of whiskey, pills, and fast food— a way of life so destructive that he's genuinely astonished that he's alive today—nearly drove him to suicide in 2008. But he overcame. Not only did he survive, but he documented every step of the journey, typing the details of his life story into his iphone, his huge thumbs padding away at his tiny screen, where the horror show of his adult existence gradually evolved into a 100-page narrative of heroic recovery. I read this unpublished memoir in utter astonishment, one of the rawest testimonies I've ever read.

Bonebreaker carries deep within him the impact of his self-directed recovery. The potential to save others informs his ambition to stay clean, to help animals, to care for his mother, to see the best in his enemies, and to serve the vulnerable. Of course, the Reeds were not burdened with the task of making such an extreme about face. Nobody in the Reed family was getting blasted on Crown Royal and methamphetamines, smashing car windows for kicks, or binging out on 12,000-calorie meals in the troughs of all-you-can-eat Chinese buffets. Bonebreaker had once done all these things for fun. The worst thing you can imagine the Reeds doing, by contrast, was maybe being late for church service.

Still, the family was trapped in a downward spiral sustained by an addictive reliance on a food system that was offering food so cheaply that they couldn't resist its allure. Bonebreaker, having recommitted himself to regular cardio and weight training, as well as officially adopting the motto "use your strength to help others," not only intuitively understood the Reed's addiction. He knew the ideal mechanism for recovery and conversion. He was convinced that he could help the Reeds escape the trap and set themselves on a path to a more meaningful life. And he also knew how to pace out that process so they would not burn out or become frustrated with results that came too slowly.

It took me a few weeks to realize something critical about Bonebreaker: He didn't have the time to help the Reeds. He was swamped, already overwhelmed trying to run his business—something he had never done before—and he was committed to training a number of other paying clients whose money he very much needed. Working over 100 hours a week, sleeping under his desk, and, sometimes, on the phone trying to delay payments to creditors, Bonebreaker's time and energy was spread thin. But he offered to help the Reeds anyway. And the Reeds agreed to be helped.

The deal was simple. Yet the deal was not simple. Bonebreaker would, for free, train the Reeds three times a week at his gym. The Reeds, in addition to attending the training sessions, would not only stick to a vegan diet, they would stick to a vegan diet as prescribed by the Engine 2 program. Heavily focused on fruits, vegetables, and whole grains,

Engine 2 is most notable for its total exclusion of added fats, including oil and non-dairy butters, and unnatural sugars (a factor relevant for Becca's diabetes). I suppose there are many diets that Bonebreaker could have prescribed, but this one, he said, "is simple and affordable and it helped me save my life." Whatever brand of veganism chosen, all that really mattered at this stage was that Engine 2 was an about face from the fast food that had long plagued the Reeds' diet.

Bonebreaker then did something that was very Bonebreaker. He invited the founder of Engine 2, and fellow Austinite, Rip Esselstyn, to come talk about his program with the Reeds. To me, this invitation seemed like a stretch. Rip speaks internationally at sold out events for big stipends. The last time I saw him in town he was having a power break-fast with Lance Armstrong. The guy, as they say, is sort of a big deal. The prospect of the famous Rip toodling over to a relatively unknown gym, located on the access road of an interstate, at the request of a person he didn't know, all in order to talk to a family he'd never heard of, seemed a little far fetched. Bonebreaker was not deterred. "What the hell," he said, "can't hurt to ask."

Rip showed up a few days later. He sat down with the Reeds, and gave them his standard talk, answering all their questions for over an hour. To punctuate the experience, Bonebreaker went out and bought the Reeds $250 worth of Engine 2 products—including oatmeal, hum-mus, salsa, and granola—before sending them home and asking them to give his offer one last thought before agreeing to commit. He wasn't going all in if they weren't going all in. They called thirty minutes later. They were in. All of them.

It was at this point in time—mid June, 2016—that Bonebreaker, who I have known for years, called me and told me about the Reed fam-ily. "You ain't going to believe this shit, brother," he said, his voice boom-ing across the line. Then he explained what he had just offered them. "You really think they'll stick with it?" I asked.

"They have no fucking choice," he said, all sweetness.

♡○♡

## THINKING BIG ABOUT BEING LESS BIG (MONTH ONE)

James and Becca began their journey toward an imagined future of wellness with respective aspirational lists scrawled on pieces of scrap paper.

Becca's went like this—
Reach 225 pounds or less (from over 350)
Feel sexy and buy an outfit at a regular store.
Have James look at me with that sparkle in his eye.
Feel better able to clean the house.
Walk five minutes straight.
Bench press 100 pounds or more.
Back fat and fat above butt—get rid of it.
Strengthen arms—flabby upper part.
Get off medication!
Ride horses on Padre Beach with James.

Be able to stand long enough to sing more than one song (church choir).

James's went like this:
**Short Term:**
Get below 250 pounds (from 290).
Feel better about myself.
Sleep.
Bench 400 pounds.
Leg press 600 pounds.
No blood pressure meds.
**Long Term:**
Weigh 210–215 pounds.
Make it to retirement.
Don't become diabetic.

The fresh zeal of a convert is something to behold. The Reeds dove into their new dietary regime with unfettered ambition. They continued to do their meal planning on Sundays, only now they planned for food they would eat at home. A typical week centered on fruit and oatmeal for breakfast, potatoes or rice and veggies for lunch, and a range of dinner options that included a veggie stir-fry (made with water instead of oil), vegan chili, veggie fajitas, bean burgers with baked sweet potato wedges, or spaghetti. Snacking was minimized; soft drinks were out of the question. Water was the beverage of choice.

James's primary concern heading into this stark dietary transition concerned taste. "I thought the food would be terrible," he said. Instead, he found himself enjoying it. What he also enjoyed was losing weight. In a couple of weeks, he dropped eleven pounds. Drew noted that his dad was coming home from work in an upbeat mood. When he said this, James dropped his chin into his chest, smiled, and bounced his head in agreement, as if he was starting to better understand his old self though the lens of the new one.

Drew was appreciating the immediacy of his own personal transition. The kitchen became his laboratory. He seemed almost relieved to have the junk food out of his diet. The control he was gradually acquiring over food preparation empowered him. He experimented widely, discovering that bell peppers and onions sautéed in a non-stick skillet, blackened and then steamed in vegetable broth, was a genius meal made perfect when served over brown rice with a side of fruit.

The family also learned how to negotiate restaurant menus. On the rare occasions—about once a week—when they went out to eat, they "veganized" their order. Unwilling to forgo their favorite sit-down place—Texican—they now skipped the queso fresco, chips, and sour cream. They ordered the veggie fajitas and corn tortillas, without the sour cream and cheese. Becca even took the step of requesting lettuce leaves to use as wraps for her veggies. On a separate occasion, when Drew went with friends to a buffalo wings restaurant called Pluckers, he settled for water and waited until he got home to eat. When his friends noticed that he wasn't eating, they felt badly, promising to consult with him before future outings. "Nobody has made fun of me," Drew told me. "My friends have been very supportive."

If the vegan transition went well from the start, the same cannot be said about the workouts. During the first gym session, Becca, who arrived in her wheelchair, was so limited in mobility that the only exercise she could reasonably perform was to walk gingerly from one side of the gym to the other. After about three minutes of back and forth, while Bonebreaker was setting Drew up on the leg press machine, Becca halted and started howling in pain. She flung herself onto a bench, moaning in agony. The furthest she had walked (in recent memory) before this workout was from her bed to the bathroom and back, so the weight of her own body, in just a matter of minutes, had caused her hip and knee to hurt so badly that she couldn't continue.

Meanwhile, at the bench press, more drama. As Bonebreaker was managing Becca's breakdown, Drew, who had just completed his three rounds of leg presses, stood up, took two steps forward, and collapsed in a heap. His legs, like the rest of his body, had lost so much strength after the gastric-bypass surgery that even light leg presses proved too much load to bear. He fell quietly, like a soft soufflé. Only James, who does manual labor during the day, seemed able to handle the workout without coming apart at the seams. He moved ably from machine to machine, doing so with workmanlike dexterity, recording every completed set in a white notebook he kept by his side. He watched his family with a look of considerable concern, but stuck to his tasks nonetheless. He was in his element.

Days later, before the second workout began, Bonebreaker asked us to gather in the gym's lobby. It was like a meeting of the Bad News Bears. Everyone voiced his or her doubts and concerns. The good news on the dietary front continued, they all agreed, but the lingering psychological aftershocks of the first workout cast a pall of discouragement over the prospects of any more gym training. This pall was darker for Becca and Drew. James stood up the whole time, notebook in hand, tugging on his grey goatee. His face, youthful and calm, looked impatient. He was ready to start the workout.

But Becca and Drew, who sat on opposite ends of a couch, looked at the door to the gym as if it was a portal to hell. They were visibly unnerved, clearly anxious about their abilities to make it through the next forty-five-minute workout. Becca glared into the gym with doubt; Drew scowled at the floor, as he often did, arms folded across his stomach in defiance, a contained and walled off young man. Mike paced and gave a pep talk. He assured them that, now that he had a baseline to work from, this day's workout would surely go better. He promised. He swore. He cajoled. But the atmosphere was tense and full of doubt.

To break the ice, I asked them how things were going at home. Drew brightened up a bit. He told me that his mother was spending more time out of her wheelchair. She was no longer texting him with food requests from the bedroom. On one occasion, he amazedly watched his mom actually step over a barrier they used to keep their dog out of the family room. "That just blew me away," he said, his eyes bright, shaking his head in mild disbelief. "I've never seen her do anything like that." Becca smiled broadly when he said this. She later told me that she and Drew were always at each other's throats—"We're too much alike," she said— and so it touched her to hear Drew talk about her in such approving terms. In any case, with this small mood uptick, we  shuffled into the workout room.

James, as he typically did, set to work with unfailing diligence, knocking out increasingly challenging sets with the only sign of effort being his reddening face, which made him look cherubic and much younger than his fifty-seven years. Becca, breathing heavily, tried walking again, only now she did so more deliberately, successfully crossing the room without pain. Her face was contorted with such intense focus that she looked as if she was walking a tight rope. When she finished, Mike had her hold onto a vertical bar with both hands and do several sets of squats. This was an exercise she enjoyed. Drew worked on his upper body and had a much better time of it. Soon, he and his dad found a rhythm together, operating in tandem, spotting and counting for each other, exchanging few words but occupying the same space with quiet, familial comfort.

But James clearly had the physical edge over Drew. The frown that etched Drew's forehead gradually deepened as it became apparent that his dad, thirty years his elder, was outpacing him in the brute strength department. When I mentioned this observation to Becca she said that, in fact, the problem went deeper than that. Before his surgery, Drew was known as "the strong guy." Everyone called him "the hoss," He was "the guy who, when you were moving from your apartment, would carry the sofa out the door on his big shoulder." But, Becca added, "He's lost that ability now and it bothers him; it hurts him; makes him feel small."

When James finished a round of bench presses, Drew reached out to help him up. James took his son's hand and Drew pulled him to a sitting position. When Drew finished his round, James reached out to reciprocate. Drew, mildly defiant, and still scowling, ignored James's hand and got up by himself, as if to say, *I don't need anyone's help, especially my old man's.*

Toward the end of the workout, Bonebreaker took Drew aside and spoke to him in private. I'm not sure what they said. When I asked, Bonebreaker brushed it off. "Everything's cool." Then he led him outside to work on his core strength. It was then that Drew, lifting a thirty-pound disk in honor of his weak core, pulled that muscle in his stomach. "How bad does it hurt?" I asked. Drew, who looked to be in miserable pain, flinched, looked at me, and in lieu of a verbal answer, waved his hand in the air as if swatting a fly.

Still, by the end of the first month, the Reeds had settled into a pattern that was yielding tangible results. All three were losing weight— with James leading the charge at nineteen pounds. But, more importantly, everyone—even Drew with his pulled muscle—was more mobile, more flexible, and more confident in his or her physical acumen. They were feeling their own limberness and restlessness. It was a good kind of restlessness, moreover, one that had them going to the neighborhood pool in the evenings rather than crowding around the television. Becca was no longer languishing in bed all day. She reiterated this point by texting me a picture of her empty bed, as if to say: *see, I'm outta there.* She was, for the first time, able to play with toys on the floor with her granddaughter, a toddler, whom she could now babysit twice a week.

On the last Monday of the first month, when I was working out with Bonebreaker (he's my trainer as well), we were puzzled to see the Reeds come into the gym. Mike pulled out his phone to check the date, making sure he wasn't supposed to train them. It wasn't a workout day for them, but they were here, as James explained, "to do some fine tuning."

During the next official workout, Becca did more squats at her vertical bar. "I'm gonna do 100 of these soon," she said. Then she turned sideways in front of the gym's full-length mirror and gave herself the once over. She turned to me. "This might be way too personal," she warned. "But the fat on my upper and lower back no longer touch." Then, with her chin held high, she walked out of the gym.

Bonebreaker waited for the Reeds to leave and reminded me in loud whisper,

"Dude! You know three weeks ago she could barely walk?"

## WEIGHT LOSS AND FREE WEIGHTS (MONTH TWO)

By July the Reeds' routine had hardened into habit. The exercise-driven positive feedback loop had sparked an endorphin rush that led them to double down on their workouts. They followed their Engine 2 program with continued devotion. Their repertoire of exercises, due to their improved mobility, expanded to include boxing, flipping tractor tires, swinging kettle bells, pedaling stationary bikes, and pulling against rowing machines. They were also happier and much chattier while working out. You could see an inner confidence rising to the surface of their outer demeanor.

Even Drew's chronic crankiness lifted considerably. His torn stomach muscle had healed and his core work, much as he disliked it, made lifting weights much easier. One day he came into the gym all smiles—rare for him—bantering with his mom and dad about them being so late all the time. With unusual excitement he told Bonebreaker and me that he had, for the first time, walked all eighteen holes of a Frisbee golf course.

He was veritably wide-eyed at his this accomplishment. For days, he had been nervous about the outing. He hadn't done anything like it since way before the surgery. But even in the 90-degree heat he motored through more competently than his thinner friends. "Man," he said, "I did it." It was the happiest I'd seen him yet. A sense of assertiveness accompanied Drew's increased energy, something that Becca was pleased to see. He'd also lost eight pounds, a real victory given that this was weight shed through his own sweat and tears rather than the normal aftereffects of gastric bypass. (Usually, at this point post surgery, patients have gained about seven pounds back.)

Later, while I was having a phone conversation with Becca, Drew walked into her room and asked her to send me a before/after pic comparing the day of his gastric bypass surgery to now. It's one of those photos where you see it and have to find a seat and say to yourself, very slowly, "holy . . . shit." The difference was striking. In the latter picture, he had a neck, shoulders, and a light smile on his face. In the former, he was bloated and miserable. It's true that much of the contrast was due to the weight lost as a result of the gastric bypass. But what seemed more important was the subtle impression of self-assuredness conveyed by the second photo. In the first pic his wore a t-shirt covered with grey skulls. In the other he sported a shirt with a Harvard "Veritas" logo and the words "Wicked" and "SMAHT."

Becca's progress continued to be remarkable. She had by now abandoned the wheelchair for good, lowered her blood sugar to normal levels (to 80 from 200), lost twenty-five pounds, and dropped three medications (one blood pressure, one insulin, and one anti-depressant). She was always eager to share her progress with me. But now I observed her sharing it with others. Her mom and dad knew all about her effort to lose weight. They had zero interest in her vegan diet (for weaklings!), but they were effusive in their praise for Becca's general attentiveness to her health. She also consulted her minister, whom she asked to pray for her. His support was similarly unconditional. Even her neurologist—whom she had to see after going off a depression drug—cheered her on. "Whatever you're doing," she said, "keep doing it."

Aside from allergies, an unavoidable dilemma in cedar-choked Austin, Becca was enjoying the physical benefits of incremental physical improvement. Even her speaking voice seemed to ring with more clarity, which seemed fitting given that she had effectively left the confinement of her bed and reentered the world. "I'm almost ready to sing," she said. "But not quite."

James also started to emerge of his shell of shyness. (Or maybe Becca was leaving him more room to talk.) Either way, he opened up with me for the first time, explaining how relaxed he was feeling, how the heat at work no longer smashed him into exhaustion, how the moral support he was getting from colleagues who were openly praising his weight loss (twenty-three pounds!) buoyed his spirits. As with Drew and Becca, his clothes were starting to make him look like he was wearing a tent. "That shirt," said Becca, motioning to the Pink Floyd sleeveless t-shirt he was wearing, "It's hanging off you, James." After a later workout he fixed his serious grey-blue eyes on me and said, "I feel the best I've felt in thirty-one years."

The atmosphere in the gym was changing in ways that further helped the Reeds stick to their mission. The rapport between Bonebreaker and the Reeds had become more intuitive and intimate. "Look into the mirror; look right at yourself, look at those lats!" he yelled at James, before turning to Becca (who was hoisting ten-pound barbells) and warning, "don't forget to breathe, mama!" as her face turned crimson red. Then he ambled over to Drew, who was struggling through a bench-press, and boomed, "hammer that shit brother!"

At other times Bonebreaker would walk around the gym and holler out whatever random tidbits of inspiration crossed his mind. "The whole family is here and they're kicking it!," he might say to the ceiling, or "people say they can't exercise, I don't care how you feel, you can always exercise!" When Bonebreaker entered these moods (usually fueled by a *lot* of caffeine), they became infectious. During one of Bonebreaker's impromptu pep talks, one that ended with the comment "oh man, you should really see me pick up a car sometime," I noticed that James and Drew, who were now actively spotting and counting for each other, would lift harder and faster, much like a runner would break into a sprint when someone cheered him on. Drew and his dad were also doing a fist bump every time they passed each other, tiny celebratory moments punctuated by Bonebreaker's staccato bombast.

All the gym-based bonhomie seemed to fuel Becca's mood, providing her with a sense of belonging to a social circle that extended beyond her family. Bonebreaker and I quietly marveled at the way she studiously worked the crowd to create an atmosphere of support, as if she knew (which she may have) that any hint of lingering negativity—the kind that dogged her when she was immobile—would sap her motivation and take her down. On many occasions, she noted how she "could not be doing this without James and Drew, and Bonebreaker and you (me)."

When she spoke like this, it always seemed like she was on the verge of waterworks. Losing weight, feeling more energized and confident, Becca was also in better touch with her emotions. She was reaching out to fellow members of the gym, many of whom took a sincere interest in the family's project. Her efforts yielded exactly the undercurrent of encouragement upon which she thrived. As always, Becca was happy to let others know what the Reeds were up to. She was proud of herself as herself; she was proud of herself as a mother and wife; and she wanted others to be proud of her in these ways, too.

One Sunday, all this support coalesced into something unexpected and sort of magical. Becca walked into the crowded gym—about eighteen people—and told Bonebreaker that today she was going to do those 100 squats. Bonebreaker, who sometimes wore sunglasses inside (his eyes got bloodshot when he fell asleep with his contacts in), flipped them to the top of his wildly tattooed head (lightning bolts) and fixed her with his soft but piercing blue eyes. "Do it, mama," he whispered.

Becca walked to the center of the gym, grabbed her pole, and started. Her mouth was set in a rictus of determination. "Breathe, mama, breathe!" Bonebreaker now shouted, as she crunched up and down. When she reached eighty squats Bonebreaker started really hyping it up, rallying others to the cause. "Twenty more! Come on! Come on, Becca!"

The gym rats walked toward Becca and formed an impromptu semicircle around her. She was now loudly huffing and puffing, struggling, about to quit. To help her, the group chanted a countdown (10-9-8 . . .). Then Becca, with a final upward thrust, hit 100. For a half second, the place was silent. Then a wave of applause filled the room. Becca's arms dropped to her side. Wiped out, she took a seat on a workout bench, hunching over in exhaustion. Then she tilted her head up to look at the people around her. She was overcome.

"Most people," she said, and then stopped herself, choked with emotion. Taking a deep breath, she tried again. "Most people…" And then broke a dam of tears and words. "Most people see a fat person like me and they run away. They don't dare talk to us. They look down on us. They think if they get near us the fat will rub off on them. But you all are so nice. Thank you for just being nice. You have no idea how it feels."

But now I think we did. James and Drew stood off to the side, a little stunned, but also quiet and proud of Becca. Bonebreaker flitted around the room handing out tissues.


## MONTH THREE: TAILORS, TRAUMA, AND CRUSHED TOES

Near the end of the third month, Becca had lost forty pounds, James about fifty, Drew about sixteen. Weight was weight—the more that came off, the better, at least for now. More importantly, though, the Reeds felt excellent. They were experiencing feelings that could not be quantified. They inhabited their bodies differently. They were, in many ways, different people than they were ninety days earlier.

The only problem involved their clothing. As Becca had observed about James's shirt, they were swimming in their shirts. Becca's covered her like a pup tent, a sartorial change she highlighted by repeatedly sending me pictures that exaggerated her overgrown outerwear. The Reeds couldn't afford to buy new clothes, especially as they planned to continue losing weight. Mike said he knew a tailor who could help them. Meanwhile, they walked around as if they were a small cult that favored flowing robes.

A better change: James now had that sparkle in his eye. It was the kind of sparkle that Becca, in her list of goals (#3), hoped to revive. Every time I saw them together James was decidedly affectionate, rubbing Becca's shoulders, or calling her "honey" and other terms of endearment, all of it a marked difference to the grumpiness he exhibited when we first met. When they talked to each other they seemed to warm into each other's presence, as if to say "I'm so happy to be talking to you at this moment even if it's about something as boring as who will get to use the car tomorrow." Drew's wry sense of humor started to express itself more freely as well. He told how me how, back in high school, he didn't participate in a single extracurricular activity but, when he learned that he could get out of class to attend yearbook photos, he snuck into every organization's photo shoot to miss class and make it look like he was Joe Senior. "I'm on practically every page of the book," he laughed.

One Sunday, the Reeds, Bonebreaker, and I went to brunch at a macrobiotic vegan restaurant in Austin. Becca wore a sundress and makeup, battling social anxiety before we entered. As we ate, I turned the conversation toward what sets people on the path toward obesity. We all agreed that, because accessible food is so awful in this country, and so cheap, obesity can just happen without one even realizing it.

But Becca and Bonebreaker were also quick to highlight something else as an underlying factor for a lot of people who lose their bodies to obesity: trauma. I knew from reading Bonebreaker's unpublished memoir (the one he wrote in the "notes" app on his phone) that, as a young man, he was hit by a truck as he walked out of a convenience store in Marlon, Texas, and never received proper medical care for his injuries. He identified this trauma as a pivotal moment in his decline. His life soon devolved into drugs, alcohol, and—linked to the drugs—violence (he sustained the permanent lump on his head after being stabbed during a fight over drugs; on another occasion he was shot in the leg, where the bullet still rests). Eating became his salvation from pain, the only thing that made him feel any better. Soon he was consuming well over 12,000 calories a day. His weight peaked at 630 pounds.

Becca's traumatic turn came earlier in life. As a young girl she was thin. A shameless tomboy, she spent a lot of time playing with boys in the neighborhood, mainly riding bikes. When she was about seven, one of the boys molested her. He touched her inappropriately and made her show her body to his friends. "You are this little girl," she told me, "and you want to belong and these were the people you hung out with; I was easily manipulated." As word spread that she was "easy" or "a slut," Becca retreated into the safety of her home. "I was afraid to leave the house. I didn't want to tell my parents. I wouldn't even go into the backyard to get on the swing set."

Eventually she did tell her parents and the boy "was banned from my yard." But still, "I didn't feel safe," she said. "All I knew was that people hurt you. They hurt you emotionally and physically." Her mom and dad worked odd shifts. They were never around enough to help Becca recover, much less fully appreciate that there was a trauma from which she had to mend. The family never had meals together, not because her parents were lazy, or neglectful, but because they had to work odd hours to make a living.

So Becca did what so many victims do: she sought recovery through food. Junk food. Sequestered in her home, she began to vegetate on the couch, watch television, and eat. Endlessly eat. A typical meal after school was several Hohos and two "ketchup sandwiches." Food, she said, "became that nurturing thing." She remembers standing in the kitchen and looking at her refrigerator and saying, "You are a fridge; you are not going to hurt me. You exist and I get something from you and you can't hurt me. You are the only thing I can get comfort from." They spent a lot of time together.

In short order, a negative feedback loop emerged. Staying inside all day made her gain weight. Gaining weight made her stay inside. The cycle, as it does for so many obese people, spun in silence. The outside world wasn't helping. In fourth grade her teacher declared open season on Becca's weight by telling her in front of the entire class that she "walked too heavy." Such insults became the norm in Becca's life at school. Over the years, disease set in—diabetes being the most worrisome. Then came arthritis. High blood pressure. And so on. Whatever narrative arc Becca might have envisioned for her life became more like a downward spiral, with very few diversions, until the summer of 2016, when she decided enough was enough and called Bonebreaker who, eight years earlier, had also undergone his own struggle. .

Becca has known James since she was fourteen. When she turned eighteen he began to show romantic interest. This was a first for Becca, who was now morbidly obese. She thought, I'm not going to miss *this* chance and starting consuming nothing but crackers and water. Obviously, she lost weight. But all James noticed was that she was getting pale and having dizzy spells and was tired all the time. "Why are you doing this to yourself?" Becca remembered him asking. "Because I want to look good for you," she said.

But James, who Becca says has never once said a mean thing to her about her body in his life, told her that he loved her for who she was and that he wanted her to stop starving herself on his behalf. They have now been married for over thirty years and they're still in love. Becca told me that, when they married, she was still uncomfortable with intimacy due to her experiences as a child. But James, she said, "was so patient. He said there was no rush about anything, and he never did pressure me once." Becca paused, and said, "He's the kindest person I know."

Becca's and James's recent doctor's visit confirmed that the changes they're making may very well promote another thirty years' of love. All of James's numbers were better. Blood pressure was down but still mildly elevated, cholesterol was way down (153 from over 200), and he had made substantial progress toward long term goal #2: avoiding diabetes. His A1C—a measure of average blood sugar, had long floated just below 7, the danger mark for diabetes. Usually it was 6.9. This time, though, it was 5.4. He was ecstatic. As for Becca, a year earlier hers had been 9.75—high enough for her doctors to tell her she'd be on insulin for the rest of her life. This time, though, she was down to 5.8. For all intents and purposes, she had reversed diabetes. Becca expected to be off all diabetes-related medications by the end of the year.

There were many more goals to check off the list, but in three months, the Reeds had made convincing progress toward doing nothing short of saving their lives.

∽○∾

If there's any good news about getting imprisoned in the food system, it's that a mere three months' of good behavior can start to get you out of it.

Nevertheless, it's the caveats of that good behavior that make the Reeds' experience instructive. It's their exception to the rule that matters.

Most notably, doing what they are doing is ridiculously difficult. The Reeds have had to alter their lives to achieve their goals. They can no longer eat, much less go near, food that they've been eating daily for thirty years. They must spend hours a week in a gym, doing exercises that only James really enjoys doing. The temptations to fall off the wagon are constant demons whispering in their ears. All three refuse to allow themselves the slightest indulgence, such as eating a bite of turkey and gravy on Thanksgiving (a meal for which they plan to arrive with their own food), or having an ice cream cone, for fear of slipping into recidivism. Finally, as the scarcity thesis reminds us, they could easily be one small mishap away from saying "screw it" and going back to junk food and the sedentary waste of their lives that have, for now, recovered.

Fate seemed intent on testing this last hypothesis. The final week of month three—and the end of my formal reporting on the Reeds— was nothing short of a horror-show. Becca had a frightening episode in which her vision blurred along with her speech. Drew noticed that something was off kilter and rushed her to the hospital. A battery of tests determined that she most likely had a mini-stroke. Four days later, she was released, but exhausted. James, for his part, slipped at work and bruised his knee badly enough to have it bandaged and kept off the ground, which meant crutches for a couple of weeks—and no workouts. Drew hyperextended his elbow while lifting weights, an injury that kept him out of the gym for a couple of weeks as well. Even Bonebreaker had a health scare, with a blood test showing signs of diabetic ketoacidosis. His doctor wanted him to come back in a few weeks. Not to be left out, I got into the mix, pulling a hamstring while running and then, in short order, breaking two toes by dropping a weight on them.

In time, we'd all recover. But, to varying degrees and in varying ways, we'd return to an existence defined by struggle. It was a struggle against a culture that wanted us to be sedentary, eating what was right in front if us, and medicating ourselves with prescribed pharmaceuticals. Given the extreme efforts to which the Reeds had gone to avoid these traps, this fight seemed wrong. It should be easier to stay on the road to health and empowerment.

One afternoon I expressed this opinion to the Reeds who, during the downtime, were working the desk at the gym to help Bonebreaker. Becca, for one, was unfazed by my doubts. She was back in the gym within a week of her incident. At the start of their transition, she reminded me that when she had listed eleven goals reversing diabetes was not one of them. When I asked her why she said, "I could never have imagined it was even possible." And then she added: "It's important to be realistic."

# CHAPTER TWO

# No Farmers, Food

There are two leading schools of thought when it comes to reforming the broken food system, the one that has trapped people such as the Reeds in the vice of bad health. One looks backwards at the supposedly simpler tactics of a pre-industrial era. Small organic farmers who raise plants and animals to serve local or specialty markets fit this bill.

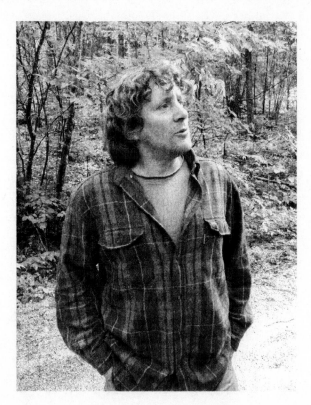

Think of Wendell Berry, who farms with horse-pulled plows on a plot of Kentucky pastoral and writes poetically about the folksy beauty of the experience. "Better than any argument," Berry has written, "is to rise at dawn and pick dew-wet red berries in a cup."

The second general approach is more futuristic. Agribusiness giants employing multi-million dollar machines to practice precision agriculture with commodity seeds, weather-predicting algorithms, and tens of thousands of employees epitomize this option. Think Monsanto. As the company's former chairman Hugh Grant once said, the "party is at Monsanto."[10] But it's a small soiree, one in which only the multinationals can attend. Dress is formal.

These two camps don't intersect. They disagree about virtually every agricultural topic on earth and (having spent time with both sides) they don't, as individuals, really even like each other very much. Their battle, however, is currently at the vital center of our discussions over food and agriculture. And that's too bad because the discussion that has emerged is unproductive. It vacillates between options that are equally limited in their ability to bring us real reform. Their dispute, call it the Food Fight, is, in the narrowness of its vision, preventing real food reform from happening. It's the main act—Wendell v. Monsanto—that should be an irrelevant sideshow.

The good news is that beyond these feuding positions, if you look far enough into the distance, there exist lesser-known but more creative actors working on food. These actors aim to take the idea of food reform to extremes that exceed the boundaries of the Food Fight. On the one hand, there are those who object to the entire idea of agriculture per se. These eccentric agricultural roustabouts are peripheral thinkers extraordinaire. Eccentric in the best possible way, they deem farming to be an unnatural and ultimately arrogant, intervention into self-sustaining ecosystems best left to their own mysterious devices. If only due to this stance alone—a thoroughgoing critique of agriculture—they have something critical to offer the world of modern agriculture.

Rejecting the entire idea that farming can be done in harmony with

---

10. http://fortune.com/2016/05/17/monsanto-ceo-feeding-planet/

nature, they choose to forage, hunt, gather, and scavenge. They humble themselves to natural systems that they never purport to fully understand. They enter nature as an acolyte enters a house of worship, humbled and awed but prepared to participate. By their very essence, these fascinating renegades reject food as the rest of us know it. That's as good a start for seeking change as any that I can imagine.

On the other end of spectrum are technophiles who aim for total agrarian control—all the way down to a plant's genetics. They see plants as machines. They understand the agricultural world in coldly technological, if not strictly atomistic, terms. Nature for them is not holistic, untouched, noble, or pristine. Nature is not natural. They enter the natural world with tools designed to conquer it in ways that make it stronger. It is a botanical library of DNA waiting to be sorted, scrambled, selected, and tinkered with in order to achieve precise results—results that bear on everything from plant yield to insect resistance to shape, color, flavor, drought resistance, texture, and nutrient density. With the technological ability to achieve in a matter of minutes what farmers historically took ten thousand years to do, these high tech tinkerers also unhinge agriculture from its traditional historical context, albeit in a very different way than the hunter-gatherers do.

They see agriculture as an endeavor that begins in the lab, continues in climate-controlled greenhouses, and culminates in legally protected patents—all before food comes to the plate. If a plant's growth could be totally removed from the vagaries of the sun, wind, soil, and rain, they'd be perfectly happy with that. No agricultural romance thrives among these pragmatic technophiles. I find this end of the spectrum just as interesting with its adherents having just as much to offer our imaginations.

These two camps similarly have fundamentally different worldviews about virtually everything. However, this opposition is, in terms of helping us think differently about food, incredibly useful. It frames conventional food production in ways that—unlike the organic/conventional, large/small, local/global, or GMO/non-GMO debates—rarely make it to the center of our ongoing dialogue about what we should eat. This neglect needs to end, because, by articulating options that exceed conventional agriculture as we know it, they are endlessly instructive in helping us to reimagine the food system we could have.

By examining these opposite extremes, I hope to start opening up a new territory of culinary thought. It would, ideally, be a territory that takes us beyond the categories that currently prevail in the dominant dialogue around how we eat. In so doing, I want to lay a broad foundation that holds within the same space the rest of this book's characters, all of whom seek some radical form of food diversity and, in turn, lay a foundation for sophisticated eating.

♡◯◑

Such an ambition especially matters for people such as the Reeds. In the previous chapter, we witnessed the Reed family struggling to rescue itself from the grasp of a food system that rendered them emotionally depressed, physically sick, and socially ostracized. The concern that lingers in the aftermath of their transition is the likely prospect of recidivism—a shameful if predictable return to square one. Statistically speaking, that'll happen. The Reeds are, according to all the research, scheduled to gain back all of their weight in the very near future. It happens to almost 90 percent of dieters in the United States. Every act of bravery you encountered in the last chapter, every ounce of fortitude and sacrifice, will, according to the numbers, likely be undone. I obviously don't want that to happen. Still, nobody should be surprised if it does.

The reason for this imminent return to the status quo is largely environmental. It's due to the offerings around us, what stocks the shelves and adorns the menus, what we wake up and, often through no choice of our own, swallow. One of the many revelations I had while following the Reeds was how the system they were fleeing constantly tried to catch up with them. I witnessed this pursuit on numerous occasions—when Becca's dad brought her greasy hash browns to eat, or when her mother cooked chicken fried steak right under her nose and taunted her to forego them, or when Bonebreaker gave permission for the family to eat some fake meats because they were getting bored with the Engine 2 regime. The Reeds resisted every time, but most mortals would not.

It was instructive to watch the Reeds stick to their regimen. The more I followed their lives, the more I came to appreciate the insidious power of the sensual lure that nagged them. And the more I was able to understand that lure, the more I was spurred to imagine a future food system that protected rather than seduced the Reeds back into their original condition. That is, the Reeds invested my own vague idea of eating promiscuously with a measure of urgency. The more I saw the idea ignored by the distracting dichotomies that shaped public discussions about food, the more I knew how was essential it was for us to talk about food in a fundamentally different way. So what follows, in light of this concern, is a comparative look at two very different ways of getting food to the table. But, again, it's a good kind of difference, a difference that takes us into new cognitive/culinary territory and expands our sense of what's possible.

These actors work from fiercely oppositional stances. And that's fine, if not completely expected. A hunter-gatherer and two agricultural biotech scientists can't be expected to see eye to eye on food. Still, the distance they create between themselves is ours to fill in with the most creative, far-flung solutions we can imagine. What we can take from their work, and the way we can combine what they offer, will set new parameters, clearing space on a wider and more inclusive table for a new and more inclusive way of eating.

## ARTHUR'S EDEN

*It was a warm mid-summer afternoon. I stood at the edge of a long pier jutting over a clear blue lake, observing the languid movements of a rainbow trout. Its colorful spectrum of scales stood lively against the slate gravel below. It's eyes black discs of anticipation. As it swam closer I crouched down for a better look. Two flicks of its tail and this fish was directly under me, transfixed with its own aquatic concerns. I took a deep, silent*

*breath and then—whoosh!—my hand shot into the water,*
*gripped the animal, which now thrashed in my hand, and pulled*
*it out. I smacked its head on the pier with a single thwap!.*
*Predator became prey. No bait, line, or net required for this*
*hunter. Just an honest meal for me to savor over a campfire.*

This was the dream I had the night before I visited Arthur Haines. In reality, I don't fish. In reality, I don't even eat fish. But the dream made sense. Arthur Haines is a modern-day hunter-gatherer. He refers to himself as a "neo-aboriginal." He's impressively built, much as you'd expect an aboriginal to be. He holds degrees in botany, one advanced, and he's an expert in the martial arts. He lives in Maine, the central part, where more people leave than come to.

I was visiting him because I wanted to better understand how a person stuck in the age of industrial food opted out of agribusiness and foraged, hunted, and fished for sustenance. I wanted to know what it took to eat as humans ate before they tamed the earth with agriculture, turned forests into fields, and local markets into food emporiums. I wanted to see what was it like to leave the culinary grid and eat an early human diet. Arthur, who promotes the neo-aboriginal lifestyle on You-Tube, was just the man.

In an attempt to score an invitation, I explained my intentions to Arthur in a series of emails (pleased that he used email). Some of my messages could have been answered faster by pony express ("oh sorry," he wrote on a couple of occasions, "I thought I had already answered you.") But in the end he generously agreed to host my visit. I do admit: part of my overall emotional disposition regarding this trip into the hinterland of Maine wasn't the best.

This whole chest-thumping subsistence act rubbed me the wrong way. Always had. Over beers with a friend in Portland the night before, I wondered if Arthur's caveman gambit was little more than macho play-acting, a tired paleo-inspired fantasy, a slightly more genuine and better-marketed approximation of our weird cultural attraction to "authentic" manhood experience, the kind achieved through self-sufficiency and a

bold suspicion of expertise. As I drove into the interior of Maine, I realized I had my own mind to open. "Be charitable today," I thought to
myself in the car, as I turned into Arthur's winding gravel driveway.

There was another concern I had about Arthur: What if he turned
out to be authentic? What if there were no affectations to filter out of
the act? Then what? I mean, could the average consumer learn anything
from Haines's Neanderthal-like meanderings? Could a neo-aboriginal
forty-two-year old with an enviable number of YouTube followers have
a meaningful lesson to offer the future of food? Or would I end up being
just a journalist making voyeuristic notations in a reporter's notebook,
chewing on medicinal roots, eliciting quotable one-liners, entertaining
Arthur's pre-packaged version of finely honed eccentricity—all in the
name of good copy? The prospect of such journalistic whoredom gutted
my dignity with small coffee spoons.

Such were my thoughts before I went to bed and had my dream
about catching a fish with my hand and banging the poor thing's head
on the pier. Strange dream. Stranger reality. In any case, I was on guard.

I showed up in a steady late-morning rainstorm. The initial scene at
Arthur's was conventional, even suburban-like, in its grey, domestic
tranquility. The house was a standard New England saltbox, yellow col-
ored, and nestled deep in a wooded, private forest. After greeting me at
the door, Arthur rejoined his partner, Nicole Leavitt, on the sofa, where
they sat together doting on their sixteen-month old daughter, Samara.
The house was dark and noiseless enough to hear a clock on the wall
tick. The couple was friendly, but, it seemed, equally guarded. We awkwardly paced around each other's motivations. Then they took me on a
tour of the house.

Nicole, whose office is in the corner of a spare bedroom that sits
off the kitchen, works at home for an insurance company. She mainly
processes disability claims, most of them diabetes related. The claims

she files, she said, are reminders of what the Standard American Diet does to human health. Haines, who grew up in Maine also eating the standard American diet (and becoming nearly diabetic as a result), now roams the forest, hunts, and conducts foraging classes from his home. Leavitt is fully supportive of the entire aboriginal food project, which she embraced with Arthur about a decade ago.

Two late-model cars were parked in a gravel patch at side of the house, a reminder that the family was, with the exception of food, notably on the grid. Beyond the gravel lot was a small hut Arthur and his friends used for processing game, which Arthur hunted with a bow and arrow. After the tour of the immediate grounds, the family removed their shoes when they re-entered the house—except for Arthur, who doesn't wear shoes in the summer. His feet are splayed out and flatted like small swimming fins. .

We went into the kitchen, which I noted had a gleaming double-door, sub-zero-like fridge. The ancient and modern interacted in the Haines compound without conflict, which seemed okay with everyone, and a reminder that Arthur's neo-aboriginal emphasis was, perhaps like the relation of his feet to the rest of his body, an exception to an otherwise (more or less) normalized situation.

Rain pattered the bay window in the kitchen. Arthur and Nicole actually started bickering about how Samara should spend the afternoon. Dad wanted her to participate in the root-gathering expedition that he was planning to take me on. Mom took a stance that struck me as decidedly non-neo-aboriginal. Concerned about the rash of insect bites across the back of Samara's neck, she wanted her to stay home, safely inside, immune from the elements, to convalesce. Mom won. Dad shook his head. Nicole treated Samara's bites with a homemade poultice that looked like yellow caulk.

It was finally agreed that we needed to eat something before heading out to forage. And it was then, at lunch, when matters started to seem more neo-aboriginal. Oddly—or maybe not so oddly considering how cavemen would have eaten—there was no obvious ritual marking the meal. Never was I provided a napkin. There was no "Let's Eat!" or "lunch is served!" announcement. Arthur simply ambled to the stove, grabbed a plate, and piled it with food—a magnificent heap of food, and dropped a clatter of utensils on the table.

He mixed wild rice that he had harvested from a local river with a scoop of soft, unpasteurized butter (bartered with a neighbor). Then he added gravy reduced from homemade bone broth, topping it off with slick cubes of venison warmed in a charred cast iron skillet. He told me he'd shot the deer the previous season with a homemade bow and obsidian-tipped arrow. He pierced the beast's chest with one hissing blow— *fssssst* —a swift and humane execution that obviated any need for farmed meat. After processing the animal in the front yard, under the hut, he canned the bounty for off-season culinary occasions such as this one. It was the first meat from a land-based animal I'd eaten in almost ten years.

Arthur hovered over his plate for a moment. I thought he was going to pray. But then, straitening his back, he angled forward and tucked in with an intensity that was feral-like. Nicole and I prepared our own plates with more deliberation. "Do you drink alcohol?" she asked me, setting down a corked bottle of mead, a fermented honey beverage that tastes like an even sweeter Riesling. In fact I do drink alcohol, even at noon when the occasion calls for it (as it will do). So did Nicole, even though she's breastfeeding and will, I assume, continue to breastfeed for many years to come.

We drank. Arthur, who was still forklifting food into his mouth, overly engaged in his food to have a sustained lunchtime conversation (and had no apparent interest in the mead), muttered while swallowing mouthful of wild rice, "Should we go out and harvest some greens?" His plate, before I'd even touched mine, was empty. The rituals of eating, for Haines, seemed to be superseded by the act's function. Nicole glanced my way and smiled in an "oh that Arthur!" way. We had just sat down. But Arthur's mind, like that of an impatient schoolboy waiting for the bell to free him from his desk, was elsewhere, probably focused on how to scavenge the next meal. His food concerns were, as I'd learn they had always been since his conversion, more about acquisition than consumption. He returned to the stove for another round.

As he did, I made a funny face at Samara, who was having the same lunch we were (and evidently always had, as mom and dad pre-chewed her meat before her baby teeth arrived). Unsure about me, this strange man in her quiet house asking a lot of questions, she looked at me and then buried her face into her mom's shoulder, leaving a patch of drool on Nicole's shirt. A few bites into lunch and I understood the reason for all that drool. The depth of flavor I encountered in Arthur's lunch tapped something elemental. My palate was experiencing some prehistoric alchemy of geology, biology, and chemistry.

It was, simply put, a spectacular lunch. The hearty food had a velvety feel and the mead sent my head into a soft whirl. My verbal reaction to the food, nothing more than a few grunts and an "oh my god that's good," became Arthur's cue to promote (read: sort of preach) the nutritional virtues of such pre-agrarian gustatory pleasure. He had me on the hook. So he leaned back and held forth while I put more lunch into my mouth, greedily eying the stove to see if seconds remained an option. I thought I knew the speech that Arthur was gearing up to deliver.

I'm well familiar with the standard critique of industrialized food. It's a critique that, in its endless iterations, is more warmed over than the lunch counter at Luby's. I know we should avoid eating grain-fed meat from animals raised in disgusting feedlots. I know we should avoid processed food laden with additives and preservatives. I even pay attention to the fruits and vegetables that the Environmental Working Group tells me are doused in corporate poison (although I think they're shameless pseudo-scientific scare-mongers, but still). I buy local, sometimes organic, sometimes uber-organic, and I try to know-my-farmer-know-my-food, as the bumper sticker instructs. I'm dubious of all the foodie bromides and I've even written a book against foodie trends. But nonetheless, perhaps hedging against my own skepticism, I very often do what the bromides instruct. Call it a culinary-version of Pascal's wager. I pretty sure my own more skeptical inclinations are correct, but just in case I'll go through the motions.

But Arthur's noontime gospel hour turned out to follow a different tune. The perils of industrial food are one thing. We know them well. But the deeper issue, Arthur explained, now gesturing at the air with his fore finger, is farming itself—yes, agriculture *per se*. Ten thousand years of it, he says, have warped us into a dangerous dependency, wreaking nutritional havoc on foods we typically call wholesome. Think your apple is the virginal product of Eden? Think again. It's a genetic bastard, spawned by that devil (agriculture), and the ultimate result of a sustained environmental assault by upstart wielders of the hoe. It's nothing close to the prehistoric tree from which it fell. Perhaps there's a reason, I thought, that when God banished Adam and Eve from the garden, he sent them to till soil.

"The produce you get at the grocery store might look nice but it's depleted," Arthur said. "Hunter gatherers ate what the land produced, not what farmers genetically sculpted, and they were healthier, taller, and almost completely cancer free. And they had better teeth." Arthur and his family appeared, indeed, to be in the possession of excellent sets of teeth.

♡○○

The house darkened as the weather worsened. I looked around to see what I could see. Forget what I said earlier about suburbia. The walls of this home were hung with handcrafted weaponry—mostly bows and arrows. The kitchen stored seasons-worth of syrup (birch and maple), desiccated fungi (chanterelles and black trumpets), a dozen mason jars of wild rice, cans of hunted venison, granulated maple sugar, and a fridge stocked with dairy products that, according to state law, couldn't leave Maine because they weren't pasteurized. The corner of the living room was stocked floor to ceiling with green five-gallon buckets of acorns. Arthur would soon grind these nuts into fine flour with a hand mill in order to make pancakes that he would serve Samara with birch syrup. No toaster waffles in the Haines-Leavitt kitchen. No toaster, actually.

You are entitled to think all the dismissive things you want to about the paleo-hipsters you may know. All those bearded Brooklynites drinking bone broth for breakfast, adding butter shots to their five dollar cups of coffee, and treating carbs as if they were kryptonite: By all means, impugn that self-absorbed tribe of over-educated oxtail eaters. But make room in your heart for an exception. Make room for Arthur. He was different.

Arthur and his clan won me over. They assuaged my skepticism. They were, in the middle of nowhere Maine, devoid of irony, replete with sincerity, and willing to put extreme culinary ideals into practice. They were doing it, moreover, with quiet, unobtrusive passion, not to mention admirable consistency. And—maybe more to the point—they were sharing it with me, a total stranger, doing so without question or doubt or obfuscation. Maybe it was the mead making me so generous, or the invigorating venison, but I was touched by the honesty of this family's neo-aboriginal meal. As with the Reeds, I found myself admiring such a radical shift to a healthier and more empowering way of life. Not to mention the underlying fortitude required to sustain it.

When I returned my attention to Arthur, he was telling a story about an argument he was having with his parents. It had been going on for months and he was on the verge of not speaking to them.

"Do you mind if I ask why?" I said.

At a family gathering, Arthur explained, "they tried to feed Samara a wheat cracker."

We went back outside after lunch and two things happened right away: The sun broke through a dense layer of clouds and Arthur's personality opened like an orchid. He talked faster, moved with elegance, made eye contact, and even smiled, thrilled to be indulging his botanical knowledge in such a lush, localized, deeply understood environment. He was a new man out in the field, a different person than the guy shifting awkwardly around a gas stove.

Liberated from domestic confinement, Arthur bounded shoeless down a canted meadow, calf muscles bulging, his cutoff army shorts riding low on his broad hips. A brook undulated like a zipper down the center of Haines's seventy-acre plot. I heard it's low cascade from the knoll where we stood. "We'll be there soon," Arthur said. "That's where wild mushrooms grow around oak trees." He took off, running down the hill like a fullback crossing the end zone.

The next two hours were exhilarating. In fact, they were unlike anything I'd ever experienced in the natural world. The brook coursed across a gently sloping hill, forming eddies in which the family swims when the weather gets warm. Arthur, as promised, moved toward the water, gesturing for me to follow. Along the way he kept bending down to introduce me to edible plants with flavors primal in intensity: Indian cucumber root, hemlock, milkweed, mustard, smartweed, sheep's earl, purslane, basswood leaves (tastes like okra), nettle, evening primrose, hog peanuts, and so on.

I loved the names and the tastes (well, most of them). I loved the textures and being outdoors around stuff I didn't even know was food. "Without place-based knowledge," Haines explained, as I chewed on a fiercely bitter medicinal root that the family used as a natural antibiotic, "we are forced into wage slavery."

I spat. Wage slavery? A little heavy handed, no?

Judging by the way we write about farming today—especially "sustainable farming"—you'd never guess *wage slavery* was the hidden truth behind the charms of the farm. From Albert Howard, the founder of organic agriculture, to Wendell Berry, the founder of poetic agriculture, to Michael Pollan, the founder of alternative agriculture, we're subjected to a different, far more bucolic narrative of agricultural virtue. A lexicon of bliss has evolved to underscore the sacred, Jeffersonian nobility of a certain kind of purity agriculture—agriculture that rejects agribusiness and follows what Howard called "Nature's rules."[11]

But Arthur doesn't agree. As he reminded me, something critical was missing in this portrayal, something that Arthur not only understood, but adjusted the entirety of his life to accommodate: There was, alas, nothing *natural*—in the strictest sense of the term—about agriculture.. It's a human construction that has existed for a blink of time, a blip of ten thousand years, less then .02 percent of the time homo sapiens have been lifting their knuckles off the ground and shuffling across for-

---

11. http://www.goodreads.com/author/quotes/1006491.Albert_Howard

est and field in search of subsistence and survival. It's as natural as your iphone is to the history of human communication.

Don't misunderstand. In that spec of time, agriculture has improved the lives of billions. But in the long term the price of admission for going agrarian has been gradual and then (with industrialization) rapid ecological catastrophe: soil depletion, climate change, over-population, dead zones in the oceans, deforestation. Agriculture, more than any other endeavor, has fueled population growth while depleting the resources that are needed to sustain that population. Again, "the worst mistake in the history of the human race," as Jared Diamond has called it. And to clarify: he wasn't talking about industrial agriculture. Just agriculture. Just growing food.

"Eating is an agricultural act," Wendell Berry has written. A fine remark. But it's also irrelevant for the vast majority of human beings who have ever eaten. Quote Berry's line to Arthur and his friend as they row through a dense thatch of wild river rice, Arthur's arms gyrating inward like windshield wipers on high speed as rice hulls clatter into the canoe, and they'll kindly beg to differ. *Agriculture?* There's nothing agricultural about *their* acts. And there's nothing agricultural about their eating patterns either. But I can assure you that their diet isn't suffering.

The distinction between Wendell and Arthur was articulated long before the arrival of industrial agriculture. In 1864, the American nature writer Charles Perkins Marsh expounded on the topic. To him, the idea of farming according to "nature's rules" was nothing short of lunacy. "Man alone is to be regarded as essentially a destructive power," he wrote, and "wherever he plants his foot, the harmonies of nature are turned to discords." That's it. Farming—even in 1864—was the latest manifestation of "artificial culture."[12] The latest hoax on nature executed by humans to help us breed, thrive, avoid starvation, and pursue other, perhaps less mercurial, endeavors.

But to an outlier such as Arthur—whom Perkins would approvingly classify as a "wandering savage"—this admonition doesn't apply. The scrappy scavenging savage "interferes comparatively little with the

---

12. McKibben (ed), *American Earth*, 74-75.

arrangements of nature," Perkins wrote. His assessment reflected how the hard-working gatherer "grows no cultivated vegetable, fells no forest, and extirpates no useful plant." The farming man, by contrast, always found himself with ecological blood on his hands: "he has felled the forests whose networks of fibrous roots bound the mould to the rocky skeleton of the earth."[13] He has conquered nature. *Felled* it. Arthur, at least as far as his food goes, opted out of that narrative; he wanted no part of our original sin. He just wanted to take care of himself and his family in a way that honored his neo-aboriginal idealism. And to an extent I can only admire, he has succeeded.

## GOCAL'S GARDEN

Six months later I got off a plane in San Diego. I walked outside into mid-morning weather so beautiful it was hard to trust it. Clear, 60 degrees, a blue sky framed by lilting palm trees, zero humidity. It was as if someone had engineered the atmosphere for a special occasion, arranging meteorological parts into a flawless whole to ensure that all concerns floated away on a Pacific breeze and the world's finest craft beer.

I sent the obligatory "I'm here!" text to my host, Dave Songstad, who was waiting for me in the airport's cell phone lot. Within minutes he zipped to the curb in his navy BMW, the older, boxier kind. His arm rested on door and he had a satisfied look on his face that said, "got it made here, dude." He leaned over to the passenger side and flashed me a thumbs up, all energy, before manually unlocking my door. I tossed my backpack to the floor, got out my notebook, and settled into the worn leather seat.

It'd been six years since I'd seen Dave. He was then working as a plant microbiologist at a satanic seed sweatshop in St. Louis. Monsanto. While he'd since put on a little weight and developed a slight limp in his step, his signature white moustache, big out-of-date glasses, and easy smile were still in evidence. Most important, he embodied the same sanguine enthusiasm I'd recalled from our first meeting, back in 2008. It was then that he took me around Monsanto for a couple of days, showing me the

---

13. Ibid., 74.

operation from bottom (where the gene sequencing machines are) to top (where the plants are grown). Never in a rush, always ready to talk about his church, jazz, his daughter's work as a budding scientist, or his latest weird lab experiment—Dave was generous with his time and knowledge.

The morning followed a delightful, if somewhat random, script. From the airport Dave took us, for reasons not entirely clear to me, to see a tree he liked (quite lovely). Then we inched down Highway 5 to La Jolla, where we walked down a hill to admire a slimy pack of seals lounging like seaside royalty on large coastal rocks as human swimmers crossed the sparkling cove between them. It gradually became evident to me that these diversions were Dave's way of showing me how pleased he was to have escaped Monsanto, where he had been stuck out in a generic St. Louis suburb, only to be settled in the weatherly paradise of southern California. When I tried to bait Dave into talking trash about his old company, he refused. "Great people," he said. "They're feeding the world over there."

♀○○

After a lunch of beans, eggs, tortillas, and salsa, Dave finally brought me to see his colleague, Greg Gocal, the man I came to interview. Gocal is an Australian. In stature he could pass as a soccer hooligan, the jovial kind who, if pushed, could turn a corner and get rough on you. He took me aside and proceeded to show off a colorful spectrum of tomatoes he was cultivating. He was so proud of his botanical handiwork it was almost endearing to witness. And indeed they were meaty, fist-sized, prideworthy specimen, streaked with those green, yellow, and red stripes, like a Clyfford Still painting, indicating *heirloom* breeds. Gocal admired them, saying, "look at that one, wow" or "oh, and let me tell you about this plant . . ."

Gocal was showing me these tomatoes on his iPad. We sat in a sterile corporate conference room, sipping black coffee from white Styrofoam cups (the coffee, I noted, was too good for the cup). We were at a firm called Cibus. Cibus, the primary reason for my visit, and the place where Dave transferred from Monsanto, is a small agricultural biotechnology company that practices an advanced genetic technique called "precision gene editing." Some critics, in a skeptical nod to the power of this technology, have called it "God's red pencil."[14]

God's red pencil was very much making sketches at the cutting edge of plant genetics. As of 2016, it was in the headline news for weeks because of a pivotal procedural breakthrough in gene editing technology called CRISPR (Clustered Regularly Interspersed Short Palindromic Repeats). With CRISPR, a protein and a "guide RNA" can now enter a plant genome and, like a programmed robot, cut DNA exactly where scientists want to cut it—something they could not previously do. MIT's Technology Review called CRISPR one of the ten most important scientific breakthroughs of 2016.

The idea of editing plant genes requires some context. For decades botanists have been able to read the DNA sequences of many plant species. This sequencing/reading literacy has helped identify the best plants to breed and hybridize in order to express specific desired traits, such as those resulting in higher yields, drought tolerance, and disease resistance. But gene editing, which is relatively new, and which Cibus practices (although it does not use CRISPR), takes matters toward greater control, precision, and speed. It enables scientists to change the DNA they sequence (and read), making the plant express exactly (rather than generally) what they wish it to say.

This is an imperfect analogy, but consider the difference between gene sequencing and editing this way: If plants were books, gene sequencing would enable us to read a bunch of volumes on say, World War II, and develop a mash-up understanding of the war. Gene editing, by contrast, would enable the reader to go into each volume and edit it to say whatever we wanted .

That of course is the rub. As you can imagine, such power understandably frightens people. Those wedded to the ebbs and flows of traditional agriculture, as well as those wary of overweening corporate power and technological abuse, fear the outcome of such a seeming ability to use "God's red pen" to scribble all over plant life. These concerns,

---

14. https://www.independentsciencenews.org/science-media/gods-red-pencil-crispr-and-the-three-myths-of-precise-genome-editing/

if sometimes overblown, are perfectly legitimate. Just as historical revisionism can be put to sinister purposes, so can botanical manipulation.

It's critical, however, that we distinguish between how a technology is being used and how it could be used. We should, of course, not seek a technological fix for every problem we stumble into or, through our greed for more, create. Such determinism, which you hear all the time from defenders of big agriculture, is as intellectually dishonest as it is prone to unintended consequences. At the same time, my training as a historian tells me that once a technology is out of the bag, it's out of the bag. Technology is inherently neutral. How it's applied can be evil, but it can also be beneficial. Gene editing is not a technology that will march backwards into obscurity because some critics fear its power. What remains to be determined is how that power will be used in the future—on what plants and for what kind of food and for whose benefit.

It's for this reason that I was reassured by Gocal's tomatoes. The hobby suggested perspective. His heirloom plants are not precision gene edited. No lab technician worked on them. They're the results of a more ancient endeavor, far distant from his vocation, which is more scientifically advanced, more removed from traditional farming patterns. Gocal understands—and is even humbled by—this distinction. His homegrown tomatoes ensure that he appreciates what's required to coax food out of the ground. Unlike a lot of heirloom tomato growers, he also knows that his endeavor thrives best on a small scale, for a small market, if not merely as a hobby.

What Gocal accomplishes as a scientist, by contrast, seeks to reach the world. Cibus, where Gocal is Senior Vice President of Research and Development, is an engineering firm with grand agricultural ambitions. It engineers—and edits—seeds on a relatively large scale. The work culture is just as different from Haines's work culture as Gocal's tomatoes are from the plants he edits. The food producers in this sterile establishment don't wear shorts and go barefoot and shoot DIY arrows at wildlife.

They wear lab coats and loafers. They squeeze pipettes and rearrange DNA. Haines, of course, would have cringed at the place. But, with all due respect to Haines, that's his problem to deal with. What was happening here at Cibus was important to the future of a diverse food system—every bit as important as what Arthur was doing back home in the woods. Perhaps even more so.

As Gocal and I continued to talk, our conversation turned from home-grown heirloom tomatoes to the lab grown plants Cibus was designing across the hall from where we sat. He became increasingly excited about explaining gene editing to me, insistent that I understand it. As he worked on me I found myself considering some basic truths that, Arthur notwithstanding, inform most of the food we eat today: You cannot separate scientists from science, you cannot separate science from crops, and thus you cannot separate crops from the scientists who made them possible. As he walked me through the mechanics of gene splicing, any lingering thoughts I had about the old family farm playing a role in the future of agriculture diminished to a fine point on the horizon of possibilities.

We like to think that nature, with the gentle assistance of the farmer, makes our food possible—that the earth's generous bounty, managed by the virtuous tiller of the soil, nurtures us. It's a comforting thought. But unless you source your food like Arthur Haines does, nature is tone deaf to your diet. So unless you plan to forage it's probably not a bad idea to accept the fact that a person in a lab coat is behind the reality of your food. Somewhere way up the food stream, peering into a microscope, there's a person with an advanced degree in the biological sciences prodding (if not outright forcing) nature to keep you well fed. Fortunately, if Cibus is any indication, these scientists are not creating so-called Frankenfood. They care deeply about what they're doing. They, too, want food with integrity. More critical for our purposes, they're doing something that's just as off the radar of traditional agriculture, just as outlier in perspective, as anything undertaken by Arthur Whereas Arthur comes at food from the outside. Cibus, seeking a better way of eating through genetics, comes at it from the inside.

Of course, that's not how we prefer to see our food, or really even want to see our food. We're emotionally attached to the earthiness of Gocal's tomatoes. Nostalgia envelops those elegant heirlooms, as well as the toilers of the soil who ushered them into existence, saved their unique seeds, and planted them through the generations, keeping the botanical past alive. We love the idea of heritage, lineage, and continuity in agriculture. We easily latch on to such simple slogans as "don't eat anything your grandmother wouldn't eat." These slogans remind us how we might one day run furrows through vegetable gardens of our own aspiration.

Point being: To appreciate deeper agricultural connections, we typically look first to nature and then to the farmer, usually the local farmer, as its interpreter. You've seen that bumper sticker: "No Farmers, No Food." That slogan matters to us—especially Americans, wedded as we are to a myth that placed yeoman farming on the frontlines of its heroic western expansion. It's an appropriate slogan for agriculture as we once knew it. It made sense when farmers—controlling seed, soil, and selection—were exclusively responsible for food production.

But Cibus suggests that those days are gone. With the world's population on the brink of 9 billion, with our understanding of plant genomes far advanced, and with the tools in place to edit plant DNA to achieve specific results, the game of traditional farming has changed. A new slogan should accompany the old one. "No scientists, No food." For better or worse, contemporary agriculture has taken a hard turn toward hard science, and with those changes, hard choices. Contemporary food production now requires that today's food rely just as readily on scientists hunched to the microscope as farmers bent to the hoe. I was at Cibus because I wanted to assess what this transition meant for the prospects of food's future. I wanted to hear what the scientists had to say about the plants that might one day broaden and diversify the human diet.

What kind of crops would the lab coats and pin striped suits at Cibus pursue? What traits would they seek? What kind of plant diversity would their technology encompass? Who would benefit the most? As with my visit to see Arthur in action, I wanted to witness the motivations behind the scientists' quest for an edited food supply. I wanted to discern what principles might someday be relevant to a newly imagined network of food. In the end, I would like some of what I heard and dislike even more  But, ultimately, I was convinced by the big argument made by Cibus: We needed to rethink food in technological terms.

Corporate scientists who tinker with plant genomes are often portrayed as lackeys who sold out to corporate greed. Corporate vultures, according to the standard narrative, highjack scientific talent with lures of endless research resources and fat salaries. Naturally, there's an element of truth to the characterization. But, to the extent that I've spoken with them, these same scientists seem to be as inherently passionate and independent minded as those working with less corporate fealty at universities. Most scientists I know are, at their core, passionate seekers of knowledge who love their work.

Gocal is a case in point. He's a trained molecular biologist with a PhD from the Australian National University. Like Dave Songstad, who is Cibus's Director of Research in cell biology, he believes that the future of food will be customized—the more precisely, the more aggressively, the better. Also like Songstad, he's perfectly comfortable blending profit-minded enterprise with responsible science. He's carefully attuned to the emotional politics of what he does. He knows very well that most critics of biotechnology don't appreciate that it would be impossible to feed millions or billions of people with his sweet patch of heirlooms. He's fascinated by the nature of this work and, like many plant biologists who tinker with genes, he wants enthusiasts of traditional agriculture to share his passion—or at least not kick it around so much.

Cibus, to this end, has something important working in its favor. What distinguishes the company from other agricultural biotech firms is that its version of cutting-edge biotechnology doesn't use transgenic modification. That is, it doesn't engineer plants that we commonly call (and deride as) GMOs—genetically modified organisms. In fact, the company says no to GMOs, a term that has become synonymous over the last twenty years with botanical corruption—or, more accurately, Dave's old company, Monsanto (aka "Monsatan"). Gocal, as with Dave, is very quick to note that there's nothing necessarily wrong with transgenic technology. "We don't see any issue with the safety of GMOs," he clarified. "But we can simply be more precise without it."

Still, this distinction between GMO and non-GMO, even if for all the wrong reasons, remains important in the court of public opinion. The GMO dispute is nothing short of a war. It has been a persistent distraction when it comes to public safety, human health, and ecological sustainability. It is a solid fact: GMOs are no more or less dangerous than conventional or organic seeds. But as many scientists concede, GMOs have also been major barriers to seeking agricultural sustainability through the benefits of biotechnology.

The opposition to GMOs, irrational or not, has been so bitter that scientists have become reluctant to pursue research that deals in any way with transgenic transfer—moving DNA from one species into another. Those who do so are frequently bullied or vilified into submission by anti-GMO activists. With fine irony, the debate has only gotten nastier as the science has become settled on the issue of GMO safety. Like a lot of deeply impassioned debates, the GMO debate is about something else. It's about something ulterior to the matter at hand, and, after ten years of following this debate, something I do not fully understand. One would reasonably think that this taint would wear off.

But it has only persisted. The fact that dozens of national and international health, science, and agriculture organizations have declared transgenic technology to be just as safe as other forms of plant breeding hardly factors into the public discussion. Neither does the FDA's claim that GMOs "are no different from naturally bred crops." Such a sober scientific message of safety—for reasons that would require volumes on scientific illiteracy, media inadequacy, and, I guess, social psychology to explain—simply hasn't registered in the public domain. In reality, the term Frankenfoods still holds persuasive power over even the most well educated consumers. Except for plant biologists. It drives them to the brink of despair, a frustration confirmed when fifty Nobel Prize winning scientists signed an official declaration of GMO safety in the summer of 2016. It confirmed their assessment that the technology was no more or less safe than conventional seed hybrids.

Perhaps there's a secure place in food's future for the mainstream acceptance of GMOs. Only time will tell on that point. But from Cibus's current perspective, the fact that the company is now free to pursue advance plant editing without the ongoing white noise of transgenic technology drowning everything else out remains critical to its work. Most notably, it suggests that whatever innovations the company pioneers (and we'll get to those) won't encounter the same wall of public (and regulatory) opposition encountered by GMOs, a wall that plant researchers at UC-Davis have angrily deemed "an obstacle to the development of new agricultural products."[15]

The emergence of non-GMO gene therapy—the kind practiced by Cibus—could certainly be a boon for the future of food. It could allow scientists to pursue a more diverse and healthier food supply without the meddling interference of anti-GMO opposition that's proven to be expert in demonizing transgenic technology for shallow political purposes. Founded in 2001, Cibus is built on a proprietary technology called Rapid Trait Development System (RTDS). The technique essentially allows scientists to do a line item edit on a plant's genetic text to select for desirable traits. I used the analogy earlier of going into a text and changing the words to make the story your own. Gocal, once we finished talking tomatoes, did one better: "It's like replacing one letter in a word with another." Again, without introducing foreign DNA, RTDS enables scientists to engineer plants to be herbicide resistant, drought resistant, disease-resistant, higher yielding, and more pliable and nutritious as a commercial food ingredient.

Just as important, Cibus is able to pursue these goals while cultivating a positive image that holds considerable cultural capital in sustainable agriculture circles. That is, it can manipulate plant genetics in

---

15. http://www.nytimes.com/2015/01/02/business/energy-environment/a-gray-area-in-regulation-of-genetically-modified-crops.html?_r=0

the lab while still being able to boast (accurately) that, even if it didn't manipulate those genes, the particular trait they seek could have theoretically appeared anyway, without direct human input. In other words, it can say with a straight face that what it does is *natural*—a point that cannot be made for most transgenic seeds. This appeal to nature might be unnecessary, an embarrassing relic of our romantic understanding of agriculture. But, again, it's also a relic that, in its appeal to public opinion, matters a lot to how the global food network will evolve in the upcoming century.

Of course any notion that what Cibus is doing is *natural* will strike many of us as totally disingenuous. But, placed in historical context, the claim does make a certain amount of sense. The attempt to achieve desirable traits by tinkering with a plant's endogenous genetic structure is exactly what ten thousand years of plant breeding has done in order to feed us. Past breeders have just accomplished the task more slowly, while wearing overalls, and with less sophisticated tools and knowledge than we now have. Unless you eat like Arthur Haines, every plant you consume looks and tastes the way it does because of this basic human quest—to produce more food in less time. In this respect, Cibus really is on an historical trajectory that's no more a diversion from mainstream agriculture than an organic farmer selling kale to locals at the farmer's market.

For whatever reason, critics of the industrial food system refuse to see it this way. To clarify its importance, though, consider the brief botanical history of, to choose just one popular global crop, the banana. Wild bananas are small, seed-studded spheres that, for all intents and purposes, are inedible. You'd rather eat a ping pong-ball stuffed with buckshot. One wayward hypothesis is that New Guineans—who appear to have domesticated the banana about 10,000 years ago—cultivated them for their hard seeds, which could be used as pellets in reed-like blowguns. Evidence here is thin. A more likely scenario is that the fat banana leaves provided shade for other cultivars, such as coffee plants, and were thereby grown as a sort of complement crop. Either way, once selective breeding led to a fleshier fruit, growers began to hybridize the banana exclusively for its edible qualities. Over thousands of years the fruit became longer, less seedy, and curved to fit the human hand—in essence a very distant cousin to the original version. To look at a banana in the supermarket today and call it natural would be to ignore this history.

As far removed as Gocal seems from traditional agriculture, he understands his work to exist within this long process of gradual adaptation to human caloric needs. He listed for me some of the products that Cibus is currently developing: Blight-resistant potatoes, herbicide-tolerant rice, wheat that results in flour that's better suited for bread baking, and canola and rapeseed that's herbicide resistant.

For those who have followed the GMO debates, "herbicide resistance" is code for "bad shit," especially among agribusiness opponents. Reliance on glyphosate—aka Roundup—for Monsanto seeds has led activists to demonize the herbicide based in part on the World Health Organization's classification of it as a "possible carcinogen" (so is coffee). But, fortunately for Cibus, the crops that it engineers to be herbicide resistant (canola namely) are designed not to resist glyphosate. Instead, they are made to resist a class of herbicides called sulfonylureas. Sulfonylureas are substantially safer than glyphosate (which is already pretty safe). The Center for Disease Control notes that sulfonylureas herbicides "have very low mammalian toxicity.[16] I wouldn't drink the stuff, but as far as herbicides go they're relatively harmless.

By the very nature of its work (and by the very nature of a word such as sulfonylureas) Cibus will inevitably strike many critics as nothing more than the latest example of Big Ag's intrusion into the corporate food system. But there's a catch with Cibus: the company is tiny. Its existence in a narrow field of biotech giants is in itself thus an empowering sign for the underdogs of the food world. The rise of Cibus suggests that there's room for small biotech companies to shape the world's future crop profile, just as there is room for small farms to play a role in a system dominated by mega-farms. Cibus employs about 100 people. Monsanto, 22,000. The non-GMO nature of Cibus's gene editing proce-

16. http://extoxnet.orst.edu/pips/primisul.htm; http://www.cdc.gov/biomonitoring/Sulfonylurea-Herbicides_BiomonitoringSummary.html;

dure, which unburdens it from the significant regulatory costs of GMOs, further allows the company to bring finely tuned seeds to growers. Much as we support small farmers, perhaps we should support small biotech firms as well. Otherwise they'll be gobbled up or driven out, much as happens with small farms.

In the current climate of sustainable agriculture, Cibus has a lot going for it. In terms of assuming a meaningful role in a future food system, it's small and versatile; it works in the realm of plant genetics but with a technology that escapes the GMO taint; it appears to take its emphasis on sustainability as more than mere lip service; it does not use glyphosate; its executives and scientists talk often about the myriad possible applications of their technology; one of their lead executives is into heirlooms.

But there's still an important question outstanding when it comes to Cibus: Does the company have any intention of capitalizing on its potential to diversify agriculture with its advanced technology? It surely could. It surely should. It has every means at its disposal to help revolutionize the standard American diet. But will it do so? It was on this very question that my initial optimism for Cibus began to sour. It is on this question, in fact, that Cibus would generally disappoint.

ᏧᎧᎤ

While sterile, the atmosphere at Cibus is also laid back and campus-like. If you were going to support your local scientist, this is where you'd go to do it. The building has a sophisticated modernist feel. Its LEED certified status—from the U. S. Green Building Council—reflects the company's touted dedication to agricultural sustainability. Behind the building are exercise rooms situated among test greenhouses, an architectural nod to the well-balanced life. The angular compound sits on a ridge overlooking a canyon where employees have spotted mountain lions lurking in the brush. In the parking lot there's a basketball court where, during my visit, lab techs shot hoops. Inside are massage chairs encouraging random moments of relaxation. You get the picture: Silicon Valley chic.

Back inside, Gocal was free-ranging across the vast conceptual landscape of plant genetics. His tone was authoritative and blunt. He leaned forward when he talked, as if to ensure that I understand exactly what he was saying. It was clear to me that his knowledge ran deep, and, while I had to ask him to parse a lot of his terminology, he was patient in doing so. But at the same time Gocal was on the defensive. His wary stance was a subtle indication that he was accustomed to being distrusted by journalists who think there's something inherently wrong with "genetic modification" of any sort.

In a pleading tone that assumed I would disagree with what he was saying, Gocal told me, "You have all this potential in plants. You have the potential to change the architecture of wheat to make it more like rice to reduce disease pressure. So why not do that?" He described Cibus's over-all mission, with unfeigned sincerity, as "gene therapy for plants." Sure, sure. I nodded. Sounded good. Really did. Then Gocal said something that really fired me up. He told me that his company's small size and flex-ible nature enabled it to think beyond agribusiness' standard row crops. "We can work in crops that are not the corn and soybeans of the world," he explained. *Now* we were getting somewhere.

Ecologically speaking, diversity-wise and promiscuity-wise, this was one of the most forward thinking observations I'd heard all day. Corn and soy, as we have seen, are at the root of everything that's wrong with industrial agriculture. It's the unsustainable crux of the animal-industrial complex. The fact that Cibus was positioned, and possibly willing, to invest beyond these bedrock agribusiness crops suggested, as much as anything else I'd heard, that the company and I may have shared a vision of a similar food future. Perhaps we saw eye to eye more than I was ever able to do with Monsanto.

But then the reality hit home. I was sitting in the offices of a cor-poration that possessed a technology capable of transforming the food system into something far more stable and diverse than we've ever imag-ined it could be. RTSD could literally rewrite the code for agriculture. But instead Cibus had to focus on turning a profit in the here and now. And it was going to do so in the safest way possible. Excited by what I was hearing from Gocal, I pushed him (perhaps unfairly) to say what I wanted him to say: That the company's signature technology could and *someday would* be deployed to diversify and fine tune the many thousands of plants we don't yet eat. But Gocal, passionate tomato grower that he was, would not say that.

I asked him to dream big with me for a bit. Talk about what could be. Think out loud about where this remarkable technology could take us. I peppered him with theoretical options about nutrient dense specialty crops. Nope. It was at this point that the high wall of reality became apparent. Local Gocal leaned back. For the first time during our conversation, he frowned.

"Flax seed," he said. *Flax seed? Seriously?* "Cibus is deeply invested in flax seed, from which Omega-3s can be extracted and incorporated into cooking oils to make them healthier." Canadian farmers were interested. Okay, fine. This step could certainly be seen as a modest move toward promiscuity. "It's a very healthy oil," Gocal stressed. *But how does it push the boundaries?* I asked. Gocal looked at me quizzically.

He then touted something called squaline, an enzyme Cibus extracted from yeast using RTDS technology. Normally harvested from the livers of sharks to be used in the cosmetics industry, squaline could now be manufactured in the lab. (*Cosmetics? Really?*) "Saving deep water sharks, that's an advantage," Gocal said. "For cosmetics companies, it's sustainable and reliable and has a purity that's just as high." Sure, yes, but, ditto my reaction to flax. Still better than corn and soy, but that's not saying much. In fact, none of this was saying much. When I pushed Gocal one more time on the plant diversity question—mentioning, say, drought resistant cow peas for African farmers, he looked at his watch to indicate that our time was up. There was work to do, squaline to synthesize, new flax seeds to design, markets to conquer.

♡☯♡

As Dave drove me to my hotel the sun was setting over downtown San Diego. It was still impossibly gorgeous outside. Healthy Californians were jogging around Balboa Park. Despite the lovely scenery, I checked in with my feelings about my Cibus experience. They were mixed. In one sense I was impressed with how honestly and deeply involved Songstad and Gocal were in their work. For these men, tinkering with genes was an impassioned affair, an endeavor they loved every bit as much as did farmers working God's green acre. We hear so much about the loyalty and virtue of the small farmer when it comes to sourcing our food. But "small scientists" embodied these qualities, too. It was evident for those who cared to visit a place such as Cibus and take a look. I really appreciated this quality, even as I wished all the expertise was leveraged to serve a better, more sustainable, more diverse purpose.

As Songstad drove, I asked him to tell me about what really excited him as a plant scientist. He became almost wistful, so enrapt in his own discussion of plant hormone research that he had to pull over his car in order to keep talking to me. Clearly, this was a man every bit as excited about food production as was Arthur Haines. But, on balance, the Cibus message left me cold. I was deflated by the stubborn lack of imagination that prevailed among the company's leaders. I was deflated by how the creative exterior failed to mirror an equally creative interior. As we passed the park full of beautiful runners I asked Dave what I kept trying to get Gocal to answer: Why won't the company branch out and bring RTSD to the strange crops that will help diversity the food system?

Why not, for example, look at something like the Svalbard Global Seed Bank and mine it for its genetic wealth and then tinker it into global usefulness? Funded by the Global Crop Diversity Trust, the seed bank holds a vast landscape of genetic diversity. Why not gene edit ancient seeds from thousands of plants in a way that could diversify the human diet on a broad scale, feeding the world, making global food justice possible, and weaning human agriculture from corn, soy, and large domesticated animals? Why not think in those terms rather than limit their work—and their imagination—to a few plants, most of which we cannot even eat?

Dave, polite and non-confrontational by nature, seemed uncomfortable with my question. He conceded that these were very interesting thoughts indeed. But we were, alas, almost to my destination. As we hit a nasty snarl of downtown traffic he hinted that it might be faster for me to get out and walk to my hotel. "I was about to suggest that," I said, and wished him the best.

Five months later I called Songstad for one last shot at the diversity question. He sighed into the phone and said, "Look, we focus on those crops (canola, rice, flax, potatoes) because we focus on business. It's a business decision. There are, in these crops, the right business driving factors. We are excited about the Canadian market, and we hope to grow in Europe, too, someday." And this was, I realized, the reality in front of us.

Fortunately, for this book, the reality in front of us is not the end, but the beginning. It's not about what's happening at the moment, but with what could be happening to revolutionize the entire idea of food and diet by using the tools we now have, honed by real people working on the fringes for a better food future.

On the surface, in the here and now, neither Arthur nor Gocal appear to have much to teach us about an accessible and revolution-ized future diet rooted in promiscuous eating. Arthur is an eccentric and somewhat incommunicative woodsman whose lifestyle is essentially impossible for a normal person to replicate. Cibus is a company that, like so many biotech companies at work today, deploys a complex and esoteric technology to promote a few cash crops that will enhance cor-porate profits while further narrowing an edible plant world that badly needs to be broadened and diversified.

But there's another way to look at this difference. Probe a little deeper into the work of Arthur and Cibus and something in their approach to food starts to seem more promising. Both Arthur and Cibus might not have much to offer in terms of what they do to acquire or produce food. But the principles guiding their pathways through the food system are essential to building an equitable, sustainable, and healthy food system of the future. Considered through the proper lens, their shared outlier status as, respectively, a hunter-gatherer and a small and independent non-GMO biotech company, provide a promising starting point for re-imagining what food could be. Their approaches are, as I see it, potentially complementary.

Arthur brings to the table an emphasis on eating the widest possible range of truly natural food, most of it plant-based, none of it from row crops (or any crops). More than any other aspect of his diet, the range and the types of foods that Arthur consumes stand out as perhaps the most instructive element of his hunter-gatherer lifestyle. The scavenging, pre-agrarian mentality thereby encourages an expansion of the human palate to include foods that consumers relying on restaurants and grocery stores have little inclination to consider. Arthur's nimble access to over 150 plants in a relatively circumscribed geographical area is a telling reminder of how desperately the rest of us constrict our diets (at our peril) to what the current food system, in its emphasis on a few foods, provides.

Cibus has a beneficial role to play as well. Despite its emphasis on a small range of not very interesting plant crops, the small biotech company has perfected a non-transgenic technique that allows scientists to read the sequenced genome of any plant and alter it to acquire a wide range of advantageous traits. Imagine taking Arthur's emphasis on diversity and combining it with Cibus's emphasis on genetic precision. Imagine drought resistant Ga Ga Hut pinto beans, flood resistant Rose Finn Apple potatoes, insect resistant Early Sprouting broccoli, and nutrient enhanced Jaune Obtuse du Doubs carrots. These are varieties you've likely never heard of, and that's the point. With the benefits conferred by gene-editing, they could become commonplace. Such rare power—God's red marker—makes it possible to grow a wider array of crops under a wider array of conditions. Bring these two foci into one—the quest for botanical diversity and the power of advanced biotechnology—and food and farming as we know it moves dramatically toward promiscuity.

I'm not especially interested in or equipped to map the policies that will get us from here to there. But I will say that much of what holds back progress centers on the narrow categories and stereotypes that shape our ideas about food and agriculture. One recurring observation I've made as a writer covering these issues is that if a person works outdoors and gets dirt under his nails to acquire food he's a hero. But if he's wearing a suit or a lab coat and meddling with seed genetics, he's a scoundrel. This dichotomy was even confirmed by the impressions that Haines and Gocal had of each other. When I told Haines that my next visit was to an agricultural biotech firm on the west coast, he looked at me as if I'd grown a set of horns. "Why would you do that?" Likewise, when I recounted my foraging experiences for Gocal, his reaction was kind of like "oh, that's very quaint and a little ridiculous." Their responses, small but telling gestures, represent the larger blinders that too often channel our thinking about food into dogma rather than creativity.

A more interesting approach to food's future requires acknowledging that both Haines and Gocal, while orbiting in different ideological and technological solar systems, are exploring contributions that, together, can take us beyond food and farming as we know it. Nobody in his right mind would suggest that the future of food should require us to make a mass transition to foraging. But we'd be foolish to ignore the message of diversity underlining Haines's approach to eating. Again, in a world where over half the plant-based calories humans eat derive from a few plants, Arthur's ability to access over a hundred nutrient dense plants, much less in this own backyard, is undeniably instructive. It's a focus that's essential to the future of food and the prospects of an optimally healthy human diet.

Now look at Greg Gocal. Nobody can reasonably advocate for the ongoing genetic modification of corn and soy that's provided the material foundation for industrial food production. Nor does it make much sense to place unbridled faith in technology as an automatic solution to anything, much less agricultural problems. But the non-GMO "gene therapy" that Cibus promotes can reasonably be interpreted as invaluable to bringing a wider array of carefully engineered plants to the human palate at affordable prices. This is as essential to the future of food as Arthur's emphasis on all natural diversity.

The biggest benefit of accepting these two seemingly disparate positions is that it clears the table for a radically different way to think about food and what it means to eat. If your emphasis is on fighting Big Ag by opposing the technologies that make Big Ag possible, you will automatically lean towards promoting solutions that favor the small farmer and "natural" agricultural methods. Likewise, if your emphasis is on dismissing the "natural," local, and slow approach to acquiring food as out of touch with a reality whereby we must feed the world, you will find yourself gravitating toward technological determinism.

But if you can transcend this unproductive dichotomy, if you can accept a framework expansive enough to include Arthur Haines and Cibus—a hunter-gatherer and a biotech company—it suddenly becomes possible to usher in outliers who point us in the direction of promiscuous eating.

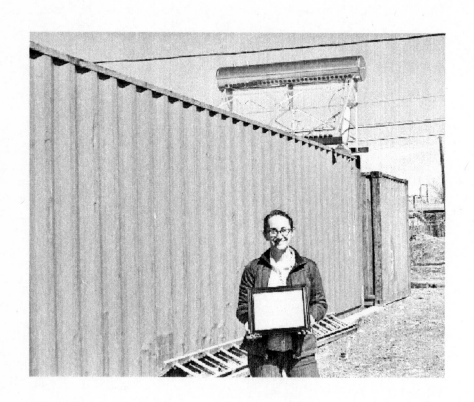

## CHAPTER THREE:

# Democratizing Protein

*"Insects all business all the time."*
—DAVID FOSTER WALLACE, *The Pale King*

*What is commonest, cheapest, nearest, easiest, is Me,*
*Me going in for my chances, spending for vast returns,*
*Adorning myself to bestow myself on the first that will take me,*
*Not asking the sky to come down to my good will,*
*Scattering it freely forever.*
—WALT WHITMAN, *Song of Myself*

On an early afternoon in April, in the blustery aftermath of an unexpected dump of snow, Daniel Asher, forty, leaned back against a sleek banquette at Denver's Linger restaurant and, prompted by the title of my book, expounded—vocally—on the connections between food and sex. His voice boomed from his chef-like frame, echoing across the dining room. "You can't just eat the same foods over and over. You have to broaden your horizons. Gotta try new things! It can't be just missionary style every time. Do all kinds of positions! Yeah, *that's good!*" He laughed.

Behind us two older women with white puffy hair shot over a look of disapproval. Asher, enrapt in developing the finer points of his sex analogy, didn't much notice or care. Plus, he was more than within his rights to air his private thoughts in the dining room of Linger: He was within his restaurant. Asher works as Linger's head chef. When it comes to preparing food, he practices what he preaches. He cooks and eats promiscuously. His current experimental preference is for a food type that Americans are, at best, ambiguous about eating: insects.

## INSECTS FOR EVERYBODY

Eating insects might not be normal in Denver—not yet anyway—but it's common throughout most of the world. Two billion people eat bugs as part of a standard diet. Many Africans and South Koreans eat locusts (grasshoppers mainly) daily, primarily after boiling and salting them. In some instances they roast insect legs and mix them with peanut butter and spices, making a savory, protein-rich spread. Mexicans harvest caterpillars from the leaves of the maguey plant and fry them into light delicacies. Queen castes of termites—which can grow to several inches in length—are popular among West Africans, especially in the Congo. In Thailand, where insects are almost a national food, street fare includes roasted water beetles, which have the size and taste of bay scallops. So they say. This list could go on for a while. But the takeaway is that, for all the squeamishness insects invoke for us at home, humans throughout the world thrive on, and deeply enjoy, an insect-based diet.[17]

A deep history underscores the human-insect connection. Hunter-gatherers, taking their cues from wild animals, couldn't have survived without eating insects. This culinary convention continued to thrive during the first complex civilizations. Romans and Greeks ate bugs. Aristotle took careful note of edible insects, writing, "The larva of the cicada on attaining full size in the ground becomes a nymph; then it tastes best, before the husk is broken. At first the males are better to eat, but after copulation the females, which are then full of white eggs." The Old Testament abounds with insect-related adulation for locusts, beetles, and grasshoppers. Native Americans, rooted to a semi-nomadic existence, normalized insects in the human diet as thoroughly as any culture on earth.[18]

---

17. https://www.si.edu/Encyclopedia_SI/nmnh/buginfo/inasfood.htm
18. http://news.nationalgeographic.com/news/2004/07/0715_040715_tvinsectfood.html

If most contemporary Americans today find the idea of eating insects off-putting, or even disgusting, Asher—who dashed to the kitchen to retrieve a pair of cricket tacos made by a sous chef—has little tolerance for that reaction. He's decidedly nonplussed by the "aw gross" response of less adventuresome eaters. He's his mother's son, and his mother, who grew up poor on a Romanian farm, served her kids, as he put it, "things like cow brain pancakes for breakfast." So the ick factor doesn't apply to Asher's palate. He expects a little more from the rest of us. Moreover, Asher believes that once consumers are eventually converted to the comforting taste of expertly prepared insect-based foods, there'll be less use for the conventional fare. Biting into his cricket tacos, I have to agree. The insects have a mild nutty taste, pleasing crunch, a sweet aftertaste, not unlike honey.

When I first met Asher he held under his arm a well-thumbed version of the book *The Third Plate* by Dan Barber. He carried it with purpose, like an evangelical minister taking scripture to the pulpit. This literary decision was, from my perspective, as favorable an omen as one could expect from an ambitious chef whom I was preparing to interview. Barber, a chef in his own right, is one of the sharpest thinkers writing about food today. He offers a vision of American cuisine miles ahead of anything else you'll find coming from today's more recognizable culinary literati. His solutions generally avoid trendiness, are doggedly pragmatic, attuned to long-term consequences, and attentive to the cultural and physical importance of good taste.

On the surface Barber might seem to be something of a food snob. But go deeper and you find that he breaks from the conventional elite food reform mentality. Notably, he argues that the "farm-to-table" movement promoted so relentlessly is ultimately limited in reach. When it comes to addressing the structural problems plaguing our food choices, the emphasis on eating local from small farmers, he suggests, doesn't necessarily address the food system's deeper problems. We can all agree that local, organic, and whole foods sourced from small farms are enjoyable luxuries with many advantages over industrial processed fare. But, as Barber explains, too often these foods require "a kind of cherry-picking of ingredients that are often ecologically demanding and expensive to grow." In other words, expensive foods that harm the environment are too often endemic to the reforms that are so popular among the foodie illuminati.

Instead of chasing after $4 peaches, as Michael Pollan infamously did (and sort of bragged about), Barber thinks we should instead strive to democratize the culinary polis. That is, we need to support an eclectic and more humble array of less precious and resource-intensive foods. He advocates offbeat but easily obtained fare such as kelp, buckwheat, barley, pea shoots, and, well, you know, fish eyeballs. ("The trick to eating a fish eyeball is to keep it in your mouth for as long as possible," writes one Chinese food blogger.)[19] Barber has cooked full meals from food waste. He approvingly quotes a chef friend of his who says, "Isn't this what it means to be a chef . . .to use what is merely half usable and make it delicious?"[20]

It's worth noting that this comment can be applied not only to professional chefs, who are best positioned to lead such an effort. But it should also apply to home cooks, regular people concerned about a just food system but, through no fault of their own, often get stuck when it comes to using the most responsible ingredients in the most diverse ways.

To Asher, Barber's question—what does it mean to be a chef?—is a much welcomed challenge. He next hustled from the kitchen with a plate of mealworm tamales for me to sample. They, too, were delicious, if a little denser than what I'm used to. The mealworm masa had a mild, earthy flavor, and it blended nicely with the soft veggies mixed inside it. The preparation and presentation were studiously simple: two soft tamales nestled together on an oval dish. No distractions, no garnish, no hyped up foodie tricks. This pared down and pragmatic arrangement highlighted another important third-plate value captured by the promise of insect cuisine: There's nothing exclusive or elitist about eating bugs.

Insects as food might seem exotic to some westerners. They might at the moment only be popular with a cohort of foodie—adventurers.

---

19. http://www.npr.org/sections/thesalt/2013/03/06/172902511/eating-eyeballs-taboo-or-tasty
20. https://www.washingtonpost.com/opinions/book-review-the-third-plate-field-notes-on-the-future-of-food-by-dan-barber/2014/07/11/61153fa0-e1f1-11e3-810f-764fe508b82d_story.html

But in fact they're the most abundant and easily acquired animals on the planet. They're a source of food that we can potentially all enjoy—an ideal, widely diversified, and underexploited food source. This democratic quality has been largely overlooked in "eat local" and "slow food" efforts to reform the food system. But it's essential to achieving comprehensive food justice. We telegraph our social values through food. If food systems are going to be grounded in bedrock principles of fairness, and if those principles are to be expressed on a global scale, they must be as close to universally achievable as possible. Right now, within the reform tradition, as Barber sometimes notes, we are nowhere close to that mark.

The sustainable food movement has directed food reform efforts for a long time. It has effectively raised awareness about the inherent dangers of the industrial food system. It has also inspired many consumers to keep fresh food moving from farm to home table rather than through restaurants, where too much cost is added and too much food is wasted. More so, in a less concrete way, the sustainable food movement stokes our sense of idealism. Who wouldn't want all our food to be "slow" and local and bursting with the benefit of freshness? And so, why not dedicate resources to nurturing the local "foodshed."

In 2009, when I delivered a more sustained critique of this movement, I underappreciated how impressively it would, to a point, scale up. In this respect it has done very well. Still, for all the appeal of localism and slow food, the advocates of these reforms routinely downplay the elephant in the room: cost. And by extension they tiptoe around the "e word": elitism. You've got to be relatively rich to sit at today's table of agricultural reform. The price of admission to eat like a locavore is an implicit agreement to eat food that costs two, three, four times more than the conventional variety. Culinary exclusivity is, by definition, expensive.

Too often our reforms fail to consider the people who are left out of this club. This unavoidable markup, and the exclusion it fosters, seems not to rest high on today's food activist agenda. Pollan, for his part, has suggested that we "pay more, eat less." Sure thing. But it's hard to imagine such advice having widespread appeal among Joe and Jane Consumer.

In this respect, the local food trend presents a tricky kind of problem for the future of food. It's one that we have yet to resolve, much less address with the proper measure of concern. What Asher is doing with insects, however, seeks to change that.

## INSECTS AND THE E WORD

To better appreciate the limitations that hamper the farm-to-table ethic, and to see the benefits of insects as an everyman's food, consider the movement's de facto headquarters—Berkeley's Chez Panisse restaurant. Chef Alice Waters's culinary mecca has been crafting meals from the freshest and most exclusive ingredients for over forty years. It's considered one of the finest dining establishments in the world. The ultimate secret to Waters's success is, above many other qualities, her abiding and uncompromising commitment to obtaining the rarest ingredients, almost of all of them regionally sourced, from the most thoughtful producers. Every review of Chez Panisse compliments this essential element of the dining experience. Reliably, it's also the first thing Waters herself will tell you about her restaurant.

One review especially captures the inner spirit of Chez Panisse. The writer began by praising the "Laughing Stock pork shoulder braised in Port wine and served with Miss Lewis's greens with house-made hot pepper vinegar." Performing a kind of kitchen kabuki act, a team of sous-chefs surrounded the restaurant's open hearth, conspicuously situated in the dining room, to slow roast and baste the pork shoulder as the audience of diners watched. The review went on to laud the "heirloom boiled black peanuts," the "Bronx grapes," and, twice, the "walnut-sized kishu tangerines." The restaurant employs a full-time "forager" to sustain working relationships with the seventy-five farms that supply the Chez Panisse enterprise with such a treasure trove of ingredients.[21] A typical meal, without wine, costs $100 per person. Including wine will easily add another $75 to the tab.

Let me be clear on something: Waters is a genius at what she does. Her vision demands acquiring a grand diversity of the finest ingredients and

---

21. http://insidescoopsf.sfgate.com/blog/2008/01/17/is-chez-panisse-overrated/

she's a virtuoso when it comes to preparing them (she has said that her other love, besides food, is architecture). She wants her patrons not only to eat well but to eat all over the map. In addition to the exclusive ingredients noted above, Waters also cooks with thyme flowers, fig leaves, rose petals, and obscure varieties of off the grid beans. It's a list that, in many ways, would make Barber proud. It's very third plate, very eating promiscuous.

But something is missing from Waters's vision: Chez Panisse is a hard club to get into. Waters may *want* access for everyone, a desire manifested in her noble effort to connect local farmers and school lunch programs. But her preferred ingredients are valuable due to their exclusivity. It is only in their exclusivity that they become appropriate for Chez Panisse. (This is especially the case for the pastured pork, which is unusually resource intensive, and thus hugely expensive, and thus very rare.) They're accessible by the few and for the few.

In and of itself, a rarified culinary experience isn't a problem. Wealthy people can eat as high on the hog as their wallet will allow (I guess). If they want to spend hundreds of dollars, and in some cases, thousands, for the indulgence of a single meal, that's their prerogative (I suppose). *But privilege shouldn't serve as a model for how food could be for the rest of us.* As much as we might want the case to be otherwise, the finest (rarest, highest quality) food the world has on offer cannot provide the foundation upon which we try to reimagine the food system for regular people.

Maybe my vision is too narrow on this point. It's true that, theoretically at least, these delicate rarities could be scaled up over time, commercialized to become more available to everyday consumers, and perhaps one day enjoyed by all. But do note that such a transition would ruin Waters's unique appeal. It would eliminate, among other qualities, the self-satisfying distinction that its diners invest in the personal cultural capital that comes from eating at Chez Panisse.

Waters has addressed this paradox by arguing that food shouldn't be so cheap. Years ago, she chastised consumers for choosing what she considered frivolous purchases over fine food. Those struggling with food bills, she said, "should make a sacrifice on the cell phone or third pair of Nike shoes." Remarkably tone deaf as this comment was, she had a point. But, as you can imagine, the advice didn't settle well within certain key demographics—such as, for starters, those who aren't rich but use cell phones, wear Nikes, and consider food prices when they shop at the grocery store or farmers' market.[22]

I hope I'm wrong, but it's hard to see an establishment as privileged and toned up as Chez Panisse introducing insects as a regular item on its menu—at least not anytime soon. It's even harder to imagine those insect offerings being made affordable to the average consumer. But the food movement, for its part, should nonetheless promote them as the kind of food source that would enable them to expand the width of its umbrella to cover more classes of people, something they repeatedly claim that they want to do. If this requires identifying less and less with places such as Chez Panisse, then so be it.

Edible insects are ideal for this role. They are diverse. They are relatively easy to raise, process, and distribute. More than any other animal product on earth, they provide a democratic and accessible protein. Given that there are hundreds of thousands of insect species, they fulfill the desire we all have for both culinary novelty and variation in taste. Finally, as far as drawing social distinctions through food goes—when it comes to the "e word"—insects are insects. Unlike with cows, pigs, or chickens, which lend themselves to a wide variation in production methods (Laughing Stock Farms vs. Hormel, for example), humble bugs don't allow a great deal of room for distinction-creating differences.

It's difficult (although, to be sure, not impossible) to envision consumers demanding locally raised crickets that were, say, humanely slaughtered (I'll get to the ethics of all this soon), or raised in high welfare conditions. But, then again, the narcissism of small differences has perpetual appeal. People who eat do some weird things.

---

22. http://www.fool.com/investing/general/2015/03/07/the-average-american-spends-this-much-on-groceries.aspx

I offer this Chez Panisse commentary to reinforce the claim that Daniel Asher, the Linger chef, may have hit a sweet spot. In his noble bid to bring insect cuisine to Denver, he is taking advantage of a protein that opinion shapers such as Waters have failed to explore within their own kitchens. He's identified a protein source that's relatively cheap and easy to produce, versatile in the kitchen, healthy (more on this soon), and ecologically responsible.

He's also done so without having to whimper on about how precious his cuisine is, how elegant and rarified his curated cornucopia has become, how the king's ransom required to dine out makes you a superior culinary being. Asher's is a more proletarian cookery. In it's best form, it's peasant food for regular people. Whether it's sourced locally, regionally, or globally, insects provide honest fare—food that leans in the direction of justice through its easy accessibility.

Plus, contrary to what so many small-scale animal farmers might fear, the transition to insect-based agriculture isn't going to drive small animal farmers off the farm and into the local welfare motel. To the contrary, insect farming has the potential to revive the small farming tradition in a way that agricultural reformers have thus far been unable to do. In Thailand, where insects are a dietary staple, 20,000 small and medium-sized farms—many owned by women—help fulfill the nation's demand. Denver, by contrast, has one insect farmer. And, as it turns out, she wouldn't mind some company.

## WENDY'S MICRO RANCH

Wendy Lu McGill is a self-confessed nerd who loves bugs. She is a PhD student at the Plant and Agrosciences Research Center at the National University of Ireland, Galway. Her dissertation, which is focused on producing insects for food, is a project she's pursuing in Denver while raising her two school-age children, who attend a local Mandarin language immersion school. Her work with insects is very local, but her outlook, and the implications of her work, is global.

Specific to her research is insect farming. It's a definite outlier endeavor. But she wants to normalize it, improving it in places where it already exists and exporting to places where it doesn't—primarily wealthier nations such as the United States. Her aim is to capitalize on the ecological and nutritional potential inherent in insect protein to improve the global food system. She'd also be perfectly happy to make a living while doing so.

McGill sees herself to be in the early phase of a corporate mission. The mission part is especially important to her. Mentally and emotionally, she's informed by her previous experience as a Peace Corp volunteer in the Ukraine. She told me:

> While during Peace Corps, I saw that food security is actually
> pretty good for most people in Ukraine, traveling and working in
> South America and Africa opened my eyes to the complexities
> of how people get enough to eat. I started researching the many
> challenges to this, and then started adding how climate change
> is, and will, affect agriculture. From this kind of dire perspective,
> farming insects for food just fit as one unusually neat solution for
> all these problems. It's certainly not THE solution, but I do think
> it's a solid one to complement others.

The contemporary environmental crisis caused in large part by traditional animal agriculture, which McGill is quick to identify and condemn, is another motivating factor. She thinks holistically about the global food system and, in so doing, envisions an integral place for insects as a replacement for the resource-consuming land animals we're overly fond of eating and urging other countries to adopt. On the other end of her mission is a better way of life for more of the world's disadvantaged people.

McGill the insect farmer is self-taught (or at least partially trained by YouTube). She's self-taught primarily because there's no one around to teach her. Professionally speaking, she's out on a limb, moving further from the trunk every day, and wondering a little obsessively about the tensile strength of where she stands. But, as of April 2016, she stands.

It's not only concerns about global poverty and ecological destruction that initially led McGill to start her farm, called Rocky Mountain Micro Ranch, in 2015. She also knew there was a ready local market for crickets and mealworms. She knew there was considerable room for more "corporate" in her mission.

Denver is an excellent place for her work. It's a culinary hotspot marked by youthful curiosity and a gig-economy ethos. It's a city that, while certainly fond of its high-end food-as-art restaurants, is on balance more amenable to ethnic dives and food carts than your average metropolis. These authentic spots dot the city. McGill is also Asher's supplier. She hand delivers to Linger ten pounds each of frozen crickets and mealworms every week, helping promote his vision of culinary promiscuity. But, as she is quick to note, she also supplies more humble food trucks.

There are over 2040 known examples of edible insects. Each has its own taste, texture, and nutritional profile. Several species are currently popular within the world's insect epicenters. These include, but are by no means limited to: locusts, mayflies, mealworms, midges, mopane worms, palm weevils, scorpions, June beetles, katydids, jewel beetles, huntsman spiders, hornworms, grasshoppers, emperor moths, earthworms, dragonflies, diving beetles, crickets, cicadas, cochineals, cactus weevils, bamboo worms, bagworms, aphids, and ants. According to one overview of edible insect diversity, "it would be nearly impossible to sample the full variety of flavours on offer in just one lifetime."

As McGill sees it, that shouldn't keep us from trying. Insects represent a vast culinary universe of taste and nutrition that we're missing out on. We're missing out on it because we're addicted to a diet of genetically homogenized chickens, pigs, and cows, resource-intensive creatures that contribute distressingly to global warming and, to boot, have the obvious cognitive and emotional ability to suffer immensely when we raise them as if they were objects for slaughter and nothing more.

The prospect of eating promiscuously, enjoying a range of tastes while ameliorating the ecological and ethical problems of conventional animal agriculture, informs McGill's deeper mission. It's an idea that she thinks could provide the foundation for a future food system capable of bringing the wealthy and poor countries of the world, not to mention the wealthy and poor people of Denver, into a tighter and more integrated culinary existence.

Insects—once they get past the "exotic" phase, once they get past the "I once ate those in Mexico City!" phase—could easily foster food justice by leveling the playing field for the culinary haves and have-nots. Perhaps one day, when there's a taco truck on every corner, the proprietors, no matter where they are from, will be handing over the counter two-dollar tacos with crickets rather than beef, mealworms rather than chicken, potato beetles rather than pork. A chicken in every pot? Boring. How about a bug in every tortilla?

## CRICKETS IN THE CAN

Trim and energetic, McGill, forty-five, has reddish-brown hair that brushes her shoulders. Sometimes she pins it up and it somehow stays in a heap behind her head. If you drew her caricature, a pair of tortoise-shell glasses perched on the bridge of her nose, and some stray springs of hair, would dominate. She has a small tattoo of two beets on her wrist. She tells me about her farm while maneuvering her car (such a sensible model I cannot remember what is was) through the snow-choked aftermath of Denver's sudden spring weather event, driving me the brief distance from Linger to the insect farm that she's in the process of building in Westwood, a decidedly rougher edge of town. When I typed "Westwood Denver" into my search engine, to see what kind of area it was, the second phrase that came up was "Westwood Denver gangs."

True to the search engine's prediction, the scene is defiantly anti-bucolic. As we arrived, McGill parallel parked with admirable expertise, somehow negotiating shoveled piles of snow as well as cars tightly situated in front and back. As I got out of her vehicle, I immediately slammed my door into the curb, apologized, squeezed out, and found myself face-to-face with a panhandler/street vendor. He was wearing a puffy brown coat and urging me to buy from him a pair of broken sunglasses for $1.50. "No Old McDonald at McGill's farm," I thought. "No, thank you, I'm good," I said to the panhandler/street vendor, as McGill searched her purse for change and tactfully suggested that I take my backpack out of the car and bring it with me..

Located in a fairly derelict lot housing a metallic tangle of retired industrial machinery, McGill's farm is accessed through a sheet metal gate secured with a thick knot of locks. We entered and crunched across a scrim of snow, the locks still jangling against the chain-link fence as we walked into the lot. From a cavernous metal warehouse on the premises emerged a young preppy-hipster-sort of guy. He was, with baby-faced energy, converting the long neglected space—it looked like an airplane hangar—into a future food co-op. He and McGill paused to talk shop. McGill, I now decided, was savvy. She had built her farm not only near a food co-op. She had also placed it adjacent to a tired plot of asphalt that somehow, under the stubborn will of another dreamer's hoe, was about to become an urban garden.

*What vision*, I thought. What faith in the sweat equity of one's younger peers. I was walking through a vacant lot of absolute urban ruination, a place evidently surrounded by gangs and outcasts, panhandlers and eye-ware hawkers, but all McGill could see was a future utopian enclave of food reformers with an insect farm anchoring it to this forlorn sprawl of urbanity.

McGill's interest in elevating insects to an industry is further supported by a desire to introduce healthier food into dietary regimes that are quickly deteriorating into diabetic disaster. Insects, again, are well situated for such a mission. Generally speaking, they are relatively low in fat, high in protein, and off the charts in micronutrients. McGill, who isn't the least prone to overstatement (she's not much of a marketer), told me, "Edible insects tend to be nutritionally dense food." Crickets, she added, "have high protein, complete amino acids, more iron than spinach, as much calcium as milk, among other micronutrients."

I would go a lot further. "Superfood" is an overused term. But if any protein source deserves the superfood designation, insects are it. Comparing equal servings of crickets and beef, crickets come out ahead on every meaningful measure. They have more protein than lean beef (33g to 22g), less fat (8g to 11g), more fiber (7.2g to 0g), and more riboflavin (34.1g to 1.8g).[23] Crickets contain three times more iron than beef, a better omega 3/6 ratio, as well as more calcium, B12, zinc, and selenium. All of these micronutrients, recall, are the ones in which even the world's wealthiest eaters have proven to be badly deficient.

Other benefits: Insects require minimal processing and are gluten free; they are wildly diverse; and they are endowed with an incredible range of flavors.[24] According to Daniella Martin, author of *Edible: An Adventure into the World of Eating Insects* (and a better marketer), bugs offer "the most efficient source of protein imaginable."

The potential environmental benefits of insect farming further motivate McGill to build an insect empire that brings insects to mass markets. Conventional animal agriculture—especially the beef industry—is an ecological horror show. As a whole, it generates over 14 percent of the world's greenhouse gas emissions, contributing more to climate change than all forms of transportation combined. Raising insects for food, by contrast, "emits almost no GHGs," as McGill wrote in an article she published in *Food Climate Research Network*.[25] If we ate insects instead of beef, pork, and chicken, greenhouse gas emissions related to agriculture would effectively disappear.

Insects convert feed into edible flesh more efficiently than any traditional farm animal. They do not require corn and soy. Water expenditures for insects are minimal. In essence, everything that's bad for large land animals is good for insects. They are better off being raised inside, with virtually no land requirements, little labor, under carefully climate-controlled conditions, in fairly high levels of concentration, and in forgotten places such as Westwood. "No one hates his job so heartily as a farmer," H.L. Mencken once wrote. But not if she farms indoors, can control the temperature, avoid droughts and floods, work comfortably during a snowstorm, and live in the big city.

23. http://www.foodandnutrition.org/September-October-2013/Are-Bugs-the-New-Beef/; http://www.the-scientist.com/?articles.view/articleNo/34172/title/Why-Insects-Should-Be-in-Your-Diet/
24. http://www.lovelivehealth.com/8-health-benefits-of-crickets/
25. http://www.fcrn.org.uk/fcrn-blogs/wendylumcgill/edible-insects-food-and-feed-farming-micro-livestock-food-security-climate

As McGill and I walked past the concrete soon-to-be urban garden, I saw in the grey distance the crimson impression of her farm. A commercial shipping container topped with thin cylindrical solar tubes, it sat amidst Denver's ashen backdrop like a New England barn on Christmas Eve—a reddish rectangle settled into a white landscape. McGill rushed toward it, as if it required immediate attention. And then, as we got closer, she asked me if I'd like to climb to the top to get a better look at the solar devices that would power the insect box.

I did not. I'm certifiably petrified of heights. But before I could decline she was extricating a metallic ladder from the crust of snow (where it had collected a sheath of ice), clanging the device to the side of the can ("this will be good for your story"), and asking if I wanted to lead the ascent. (*No. No. No.*) The ladder did not look well. It looked like it had been beaten up. But, head down, breath held, I climbed. A cold wind whipped around me as I summited the can, tottering on top before falling to my hands and knees, shaking, then recovering myself and cavalierly holding the ladder steady for McGill to scale, which she did as if she was stepping on a stool to grab something off the top shelf of the pantry. We made it.

I stood on tottering legs and focused. And there they were. These slender photovoltaic tubes—about twenty-five of them aligned together on the roof at a 45-degree angle— served as tangible reminders that what was taking place in the box below was far from frivolous. Perhaps it really did have profound agricultural significance. The red can was a solemn promise that this project would achieve the elusive goal of producing ample quantities of healthy animal flesh under conditions that, possibly, for once, could accurately be called a word that has been uttered to the point of meaninglessness: *sustainable.* Here, in these tubes, was the "mission" part of corporate mission. McGill was reclaiming the idea of sustainable.

This distinction may seem peripheral, but it's in fact central to the future of food. Many of the "sustainable" alternatives to industrial animal agriculture—pastured chickens, grass-fed beef, and free-range pork raised on small farms, and what not—are obviously improvements on the industrial model. But, especially when compared to the insect farm, they cannot, in all fairness to the term, be called sustainable.

They are saddled with too many environmental and ethical setbacks. Some agricultural facts go unmentioned. But here is what the sustainable agriculture advocates aren't talking about: Grass-fed beef actually produces more greenhouse gasses than conventional corn fed cows. Chickens raised on pasture suffer higher rates of predation—and premature death—than those that are confined. Pigs that are free-ranged must have their noses mutilated with rings to prevent rooting—a device that makes the pig's nose hurt every time it touches the ground. Pastured pigs also produce more phosphorous in their manure than their crated counterparts. In some studies, pastured eggs have had higher rates of salmonella than confined ones. Insect agriculture has the potential to be an alternative to these alternatives.

So, boldly atop the can, staring at downtown Denver to the east, I had the warm feeling that perhaps there was something new under the sun. Maybe I was standing on top of a game changer for the food system. So much of what McGill was doing with this project made very good sense. The arguments for this nascent agricultural endeavor have been made and they were, as far as I could tell, convincing. The media has embraced the idea, too, with dozens of optimistic articles running in high-end publications, all praising the prospects of edible insects. The word "entomophagy"—eating insects—isn't nearly as foreign as it once was. Even the World Health Organization recently endorsed the mass production and consumption of insects, justifying their move on ecological and health-related grounds.

It also occurred to me that McGill was defining a building block that was easily replicable. This lone red can, which once carried who knows what-all from China, represented the starting point of a decentralized industry run not by a huge corporate conglomerate, but by a graduate student who could afford a $4000 container, some food-grade crickets, a source of heat, and some growing bins from the Container Store. As McGill is the first to admit, if she can do this, anyone can.

And then there's the sheer volume produced. McGill estimates that, inside her container, she will, without hiring help, raise up to 200,000 crickets at a time—a quantity that amounts to approximately 150 pounds of cricket meat a month. That's over a ton of flesh grown annually on a plot of land smaller than a food truck (about 320 square feet). To put this quantity in perspective, consider beef. A typical grass fed cow—the popular alternative to corn-raised beef—takes fourteen months to reach slaughter weight and would need at least ten acres of land to fatten up. At the end of the day it might yield 450 pounds of trimmed beef. That's half the edible flesh, less healthy edible flesh, produced on 1,450 times more land.

When it comes to the question of sustainability, it's no comparison. In terms of density of production, a rubric that, according to some experts, is the most important ecological concept food producers can pursue, there's no choice. And if the idea of missing out on burgers is a nightmare, there happens to be such a thing as a cricket burger.

♡O○

As of April of 2016, all the optimism surrounding McGill's insect endeavor was tempered by an important caveat: There were as yet no bugs in the can. When I finally alighted back on earth and entered the metallic farm, it became quickly evident that there were a grand total of zero insects under incubation. "The damn shelves need to be put in," McGill said, hands on her hips, toeing the linoleum floor in mild frustration. "Well, shit."

She was referring to those latticed metal shelves popular in professional kitchens. She'd ordered them from a kitchen supply company weeks ago. They'd never arrived. Fights over the phone had ensued with the manager; despair had set in; angry emails crisscrossed in cyberspace. It was on those shelves that she planned to stack her insect pods. "They should be here any day," she said. "Or maybe some day." Another expletive. "Maybe never."

I did note that, on the bright side, the solar tubes were not only very attractive they but were working splendidly. It was hot and humid inside the empty container. "Feels like Costa Rica," I observed. Still, contemplating the possibility that I'd just flown to Denver to risk my life atop an icy farm-can only to encounter a vacant shipping canister, I asked after the inventory. Where were the bugs? "About that," she said. "Back to the car." Within fifteen minutes we pulled up in front of McGill's modest, yellow, shingled, single-family home. A dozen oversized rectangular boxes fanned across the yard like a monstrous spread of cards. "Shelving!".

McGill's father—a stage actor who has appeared in shows such as *Law and Order* and *The Sopranos* stood next to her two young kids, a boy and a girl, aged eight and ten. They had rushed out the door when they saw McGill's car, eyes filled with excitement, pointing to the large boxes. "They came!" said McGill's dad, who was already bent to the task of stacking the unwieldy boxes upright. He said he'd help her move them to the red can right away. McGill promptly ordered him to put the things down, motioning to his seventy-two-year old back. She had a friend, with a truck, who would help out.

"I'm here to see the insects," I said to the kids.

"They smell gross," said one.

"They smell terrible," said the other.

"They smell *earthy*," McGill corrected them.

I followed McGill and her two large white dogs down a flight of stairs to the basement. It immediately became evident to me that smell was indeed an issue. It was somewhere in between the three assessments. Not gross. Not terrible. But not quite *earthy* either. There was a waft of funkiness in the air. The crickets and mealworms were housed in cages like the ones used to contain a pet snake or lizard. They lined the walls at waist level, one after the other, around the entire room. .

I browsed over the confined creatures like a patron passing through an art gallery, observing a monotony of skittering crickets and lazing mealworms. My thoughts turned to sentience. I momentarily considered them as living beings while, at the same time, categorizing them as not very significant living beings. They were twitching masses of ganglia, morally irrelevant lumps of cellular arrangements. Fruits of the earth. Senseless. Stupid. Shitty. Stinking. Bugs. All these descriptions sounded about right.

Or so I told myself.

## A NECESSARY DETOUR INTO A LONGISH ARGUMENT THAT WILL BUG VEGANS

Whenever we talk about eating animals we also have to talk about ethics. Technically speaking, insect farming demands incessant murder. In the corner of the basement, just across from the breeding cages, stood McGill's means of execution: a large white deep freeze. It hummed with quiet sadism. McGill would never call herself the matron of an abattoir. But the fact remained that she killed hundreds of thousands of animals every month— by freezing them, slowly and without their consent, in this icy death chamber.

McGill acknowledged the truly massive extent of the slaughter. She confessed to being "a person who dispatches tens of thousands of souls regularly to a frozen death and who aspires to increase that number significantly." Of course, the killing is hardly a problem in and of itself. But if the killing is unnecessary, and the animals are sentient, and we're freezing them to death, slowly, we have, if not blood, then at least a moral issue on our hands. So, for this very reason, the question that I didn't want to address—although I knew I had to address it—was one that may be the most morally significant for the future of insect food. *Could these skittering things suffer?*

Did they experience pain or, as I intuited, did they just thoughtlessly twitch, as if their limbs jerked by neurological remote control? By promoting eating insects am I unwittingly endorsing (and McGill carrying out) a never-ending holocaust of critters that could, however nominally, be deemed sentient? Was McGill's admitted anxiety over the potential soulful nature of insects—an anxiety I wish she didn't possess—in any way justified by the empirical reality of suffering?

Grappling with this question might seem like a joke. But it's not. I treat the matter of insect death, and animal suffering in general, as a profoundly serious ethical concern. And because I see absolutely no point in imagining an exemplary future food system if it ends up ignoring the reality of animal suffering, I felt obligated to face this issue as honestly as I could. And, truth be told, I was not much comforted by the most honest general answer I could find to the prospect of insect sentience:

unlikely but possible. Of course, "it's possible" is just another way of saying "we'll never know." But that's okay, because it's within that ambiguity— between the "it's possible" and "we'll never know"—that we can start to do some important legwork on the question of insect suffering.

Some good news for the prospects of ethical insect food first: In so far as we agree to produce and consume insects, we can dramatically reduce the suffering we intentionally cause to obviously sentient creatures. Killing ten billion land animals a year (which we now do in the United States)—*all of whom we know for certain to have a sense of self and a deep capacity for suffering*—is a significant, if not the single most significant, mark against the contemporary food system. Insects could dramatically ameliorate this suffering. It therefore seems perfectly sensible to promote a system that could end the vast majority of animal agriculture as we know it. And it seems even more sensible if we do this by replacing animals that obviously suffer with those that *might suffer*— and, perhaps, probably don't suffer—in our diet. Hence: the potentially legitimate place of insects in the future food system.

This is not, from a purely ethical perspective, an ideal position to hold. A vocal minority of ethical eaters disagrees intensely with killing insects in light of the unsettled question of their sentience. Vegans most notably reject the argument for replacing traditional animal agriculture with commercial insect production. They want all animal exploitation to end. On the surface, their reason is simple enough. Vegans don't eat animals; insects are animals; vegans therefore don't eat insects. Case closed.

But beneath the surface, this convenient syllogism obscures more than it clarifies. It overlooks the very real possibility that vegans, by virtue of their otherwise admirable quest to reduce animal suffering, may not only be morally *permitted* to eat insects; they may actually be *obligated* to do so in order to adhere to their ideals. In fact, after a lot of thought, I've concluded this to be the case. What follows is therefore my argument for why vegans are ethically compelled, even in light of the ambiguity surrounding insect sentience, to eat bugs.

♡○○

The argument begins with an agricultural reality we seldom acknowl-edge: the number of sentient animals killed to grow and harvest edible plants. Farmers routinely unleash an arsenal of agricultural weaponry upon unquestionably sentient "pests"—squirrels, rabbits, mice, moles, voles, deer, wolves, and coyote—who compete for our plant crops. Esti-mates are that about fifty-five sentient animals are killed to produce 220 pounds of wheat.[26]  Come harvest time, combines and harvesters unavoidably shred millions of self-aware critters lurking among the crops into a gory oblivion.

The suffering that's required to bring seemingly "humane" plant foods to our plate is thereby almost as palpable perhaps as the suffering of those animals slaughtered to feed us chicken, pork, and beef. If you want to play the numbers game on this point, be prepared to confront a hard fact: There is more suffering required to produce plants than to raise large animals on grass and eat them in lieu of more plants. Anyone who thinks that growing plants for food is *ipso facto* kinder to animals doesn't know much about agriculture, much less what it might feel like to get sliced by a combine or choked into asphyxiation by a rodenticide. Absurd as the idea seems, a vegan would personally do less harm to ani-mals by subsisting off a large animal or two every year—like the Inuit do with seals—than eating plants.

The violent agricultural reality behind plant production isn't neces-sarily the vegan's problem. To the extent that they address this problem, vegans respond that incidental animal deaths caused from growing kale and carrots and sweet corn are ethically preferable to directly killing ani-mals to eat bacon and pork. There's something to that argument. This response, moreover, carries added weight when it's complemented with genuine efforts to improve agriculture in order to minimize rates of inci-dental death, which many farmers do. There's such a thing, for example, as veganic agriculture—farming in a way that attempts to reduce animal suffering by avoiding all soil amendments that contain animals by-prod-ucts such as bone and bloodmeal, avoiding all pesticides, and sometimes trying to remove rodents manually or even building enclosures around

---

26. http://theconversation.com/ordering-the-vegetarian-meal-theres-more-animal-blood-on-your-hands-4659

crops. Modest gains have been achieved through these efforts. But, all things considered, it's hard to imagine growing a commercial amount of food, at least at this point in time, without killing a lot of animals.

All that said, with the insect option now on the table, the vegan equation has fundamentally changed. The choice is no longer between the incidental or non-incidental deaths of obviously sentient creatures. It's no longer between mice crushed by a combine or pigs taken to the abattoir. Instead, with insects now in the mix, it's between the intentional death of animals that most likely suffer minimally or maybe even not at all (insects) and those that we know for sure suffer terribly (bunnies, deer, mice, etc.) when plants are grown for food.

This choice places the ethical vegan in a bind. It makes it far more difficult to reconcile the vegan's defining mission—to reduce animal harm —with an exclusively plant-based diet. After all, the more that vegans replaced plant-based calories with insect-based calories, the fewer animals they'd end up harming. One response to this dilemma is to dismiss it outright. Just declare and insist that insects are sentient creatures, that they can suffer as much as any other animal we eat, and leave it at that.

But there's simply not enough evidence to make this move. While the question of insect sentience has produced a minefield of disagreement among scientists and philosophers, even the most dogged supporters of the proposition (such as Jeffrey Lockwood, an entomologist who instructs his graduate students to anesthetize insects before experimenting on them) concede that there's zero hard evidence to support the prospect of insect suffering. In the end, after all the theorizing, there's still ample room to doubt the presence of sentience when it comes to insects. By contrast, there is absolutely no room for such doubt when it comes to the mammals and birds killed in agriculture.

Other entomologists insist that the idea of insect suffering is complete lunacy. Hans Smid, of Wageningen University in the Netherlands, is an expert on the brains of parasitic wasps. These wasps are some of the most behaviorally sophisticated insects on Earth. "I am absolutely convinced," he told the *Washington Post* "that insects do not feel pain." The prospect of insect sentience also makes little evolutionary sense. Robert

Elwood, a professor of the biological sciences at Queens University in Belfast, notes that the capacity to suffer would provide insects no survival advantage. "From an evolutionary perspective," he told the Post, "the only reason for pain that makes sense to me is that it enables long-term protection."

But insects don't live long-term lives. The average lifespan of a field cricket is five to six weeks. Self-protection for insects, in essence, comes not from drawing on a stored bank of memories. It has no need for a history of painful and pleasurable experiences, the kind that are managed to maintain a sense of self. This wouldn't make sense for such a short life span. Rather insect self-protection derives from remarkable reproductive efficiency, a capacity that obviates any need to learn from past mistakes—just make new creatures. What memory and consciousness accomplish for some species, reproductive efficiency does for others. Arguably, not only is sentience not evident in insects, but the deliberation that it demands could be a detriment to insect survival.

Of course the vegan could, at this point, throw down the precautionary card. He could say that, because there is *some* disagreement, it's better to be on the safe side and not raise insects for food at all. But this, too, would be disingenuous. The little confusion that does exist must be weighed against the known competing moral consideration: Those untold numbers of vertebrates that unquestionably suffer when plants are grown for people to eat. If vegans who are unsure that insects suffer take the leap and eat insects anyway, they know there's a slim chance the animals they eat might suffer. If they stick to an exclusive plant-based diet, they must concede that animals will definitely suffer.

To carry this argument one final step further, even if one believes, based on flimsy evidence, that insects definitely suffer, then there is still the manner of insect death to consider. It could, if properly administered, be far less painful than the death experienced by fuzzy little mammals ground up by harvesters and gutted by rodenticides. When a fly is swatted with a clean hit, for example, death is so mercifully swift and definitive that it's virtually imperceptible to the critter. (As for the slow freeze, well, maybe not so much).

Critics might object that, even if the death is instant, an insect has a theoretical right to the rest of its life. But it would be hard to find a rational person to make such a case. For the field mice, much less the pig or cow, for whom botched slaughters are routine, the rational person would surely concede that the death is much worse. At some point, common sense must enter into these important deliberations.

Insect farmers such as McGill harvest their animals for slaughter at the very end of the animal's natural life—again, about five weeks for crickets. A cow, pig, or chicken, by contrast, is slaughtered after having lived only a small fraction of its natural life span, maybe 20 percent of it. This point strongly mitigates against the claim that the insect has some sort of right to the remainder of its life, which may be only a few days. Considering all these factors, if the goal is to reduce suffering, the choice seems unavoidable: Vegans should eat insects. Indeed, we all should.

## THE INTOXICATING SMELL OF RESPONSIBLE FEED

The final bit of evidence tipping the scales toward my resolution to become a moral cheerleader for insects was the nature of their feed. Conventional animal agriculture demands that hundreds of millions of acres be dedicated toward producing externally sourced feed. Every day, a single industrial beef cow needs about twenty-four pounds of corn-based food. This food, for a single cow's life, is grown on a patch of land the size of a hundred football fields. That patch looks nice from the highway, clean and angular from the sky. But from those bucolic plots of grain ensue complete ecological mayhem.

More than a third of all arable land in the United States is sacrificed to grow the crops that make this animal food. The majority of insecticides sprayed in the U.S. are sprayed to grow this meal. In addition to alfalfa—another livestock expenditure—this meal accounts for most of the agricultural water usage in the United States, as well as for the vast majority of fertilizer, from which nitrogen leaches off into the Gulf of Mexico and creates capacious dead zones. More animals—insects included—are killed growing corn and soy than for any other industrial agricultural product on the planet. And, despite all these costs, only about 40 percent of all the feed we produce gets turned into edible flesh. The movement of land animals burned calories, and more calories go to building sense animal bones than edible flesh. It is, in short, an absolutely lunatic calculation, possibly the dumbest misallocation of natural resources in human history.

Insects convert the entirety of what they eat into edible flesh, and that edible flesh is, unlike farmed animals with bones, the entire creature. To reinforce how differently the feed situation is in insect agriculture, McGill completed my tour by taking me to the last link in the day's production chain: Wit's End Brewing.

It's the kind of microbrewery commonly tucked into pseudo-gentrified locations of urban centers throughout the country. This one was situated in an alley lined by a row of loading docks. A black chalkboard listed craft beers on tap. Under it, a burly guy in rubber boots read gauges on industrial-sized silver brewing vats. A tap keeper with the obligatory brewing beard and Buddy Holly glasses approached. When he saw it was Wendy, he lit up. The two discussed a collaboration I wasn't supposed to hear about (something about a cricket beer I think) before the brewer started pouring generous samples of his latest fermentations into shot-sized glassware.

We eventually ordered pints of thick stouts, reviewed my notes from the day, and discussed the finer points of insect farming (feed conversion, FDA regulation, stuff). On the way out of the brewery, the real reason for McGill's foray to Wit's End—and the part that nicely wraps up my feed argument— became clear. McGill took out two buckets and a hand shovel from the back of her car, headed over to a large white barrel to the right of the brewery, and, with several satisfying scooping sounds, filled her containers with spent brewers grain. It looked and smelled like toasty, whole grain oatmeal. "My feed source," she said.

Better than the Iowa landscape, I thought.

## A GREY CAN IN A BLACK CAN IN A RED CAN—IN A NEW PLACE

McGill is her own harshest critic. Reflecting on her start-up experience, she declared herself to be "naïve-stupid" in many ways. For the record, she's prone to self-deprecation, and is neither naïve nor stupid, much less any combo of the two. But like any mission-oriented business mired in the innocence of infancy, Rocky Mountain Micro Ranch suffered some early growing pains. A short list of the teachable moments, according to McGill, include the following:

a) Her "corporate mission" initially put more emphasis into the "mission" than the "corporate"—she was, in essence, thinking too much like a George Soros and not enough like Gordon Gecko.

b) McGill placed too much trust in some Finland consultants who for too long offered her bad advice (or no advice) that she assumed was just normal behavior and forgave their uselessness (see a).

c) She missed some zoning fine print rules that endangered her space at the co-op (see a,b).

d) She hadn't pursued profitable and productive collaborations within her own industry—she had not "networked" enough (see all of the above).

In September I had another chance to meet McGill in Denver. I was anxious to see how she addressed these concerns. Turns out much had changed. Some important developments helped foster her final push to reach a steadier market. It was a market that, as if to heighten her resolve, kept knocking on her door asking for increasingly larger quantities of insects that, alas, she could not immediately provide. This inability made for an intolerable state of corporate-mission existence. Rearing her corporate head a little more than usual, testing her business mettle in the breach, she determined that this situation needed better focus.

To that end, between April and September, McGill did the following:

a) Attended the first annual U.S. insect producers' conference in Detroit.

b) Got a forty-pound order she could neither meet nor refuse.

c) Was unceremoniously booted from her vacant lot/future food co-op due to some obscure code violation that she missed.

d) Discovered that a Sacramento tech firm had something to offer a lone insect farmer in Denver.

As near as I could tell, the common thread running through all these factors, and what eventually knitted the operation into whole cloth, was McGill's explicit decision to start thinking more like a company. "I sound like a business person," she said, after discussing with me some of her marketing strategies. She added, bemusedly, "I have spreadsheets." And how did she feel about that?

"Ugh but yay."

"Eating Insects Detroit 2016"—as the conference was billed—was a pivotal weekend for McGill. The event actually required security detail. Some seemingly madman biologist who had been ranting online about how certain cricket flour manufacturers had stolen his mint-worthy ideas had registered to attend. (This guy had once contacted *me* about an article I'd written in a magazine about edible insects—and, indeed, I will attest: he was an extraordinary ranter). Due to the semi-unhinged nature of his social media missives, many of which vaguely hinted at some manner of revenge, the conference host, Wayne State University, thought it best to hire some backup brass. As promised, the mad scientist showed up. And, as McGill explained, he turned out to be a total sweetheart. "He was the nicest guy you'd ever met. He came out and drank beers with us," she said. "I think he just needed to be around people."

"He needed a hug," I said.

"He needed a hug," she agreed.

Being around such people served McGill well, too. When I spoke to her about the conference (I was planning to attend it, too, but my flight was cancelled and my rebooking would have put me in too late to justify the cost), she said she pretty much didn't sleep much in Detroit. Thrilled by the chance to meet so many people working in her element, enamored that every facet of this collective start-up industry was represented, and being an inherently gregarious sort of person, McGill shifted into schmooze mode. She talked and she listened and her network of contacts expanded.

The outcome was a series of connections with people more knowledgeable about what she was doing than she was. Her correspondence with these new associates made the limb she was out on feel much more secure. Or, as she now put it, "I now felt less stupid naïve."

Particularly notable in terms of production capacity was the connection she forged with company called Bitwater Farms. This is a fascinating tech-oriented agricultural operation dedicated to helping small farmers waste less but produce more—often with cutting edge, niche-oriented solutions. Their online promotional brochure claims that its researchers have "cracked the code" for how farmers could grow insects—which they call "a crop"—"safely and efficiently."[27] Over a double espresso (mine) and cup of iced tea (hers) at a paleo-themed coffee bar in Denver, McGill explained the nature of that code in preparation for us going to see it at work. (She also marketed her crickets to the owner of the Paleo coffee shop, who balked because his wife was allergic to shellfish.)

Bitwater provided McGill "a system to test." Interestingly—and appropriately, given that McGill lives in Colorado—the system was based on indoor plant growth of, mainly marijuana. The biggest challenge faced by McGill inside her insect can was monitoring temperature and keeping humidity constant. This challenge was one that Bitwater

27. http://www.bitwaterfarms.com/about/

noticed she shared with greenhouse managers, as well as pot growers, and so the Bitwater guys went to work.

Through an elegant example of technology transfer, Bitwater farms introduced McGill to square-shaped black Mylar-lined tents—again, the kind often used by advanced pot growers. They advised her to equip the inside with a small humidifier and a space heater, devices that would make the black box within the red box feel like a tropical rainforest. Insects—in this case crickets—would thrive inside grey plastic boxes under the output of Home Depot-sourced machines.

As for the grey boxes, Bitwater advised McGill to adopt opaque containers for cricket housing. The previous cages used a top screen for ventilation. But airflow was poor; the light too intense; insects prematurely expired too rapidly. For ventilation in the new containers, Bitwater suggested that McGill carve holes in the plastic bins and fit into them little tea-strainer screens. These grey bins marked with little screen bulges were stacked inside the black tent, which was sitting inside the red can. The whole arrangement was taking on the appearance of a large Russian doll. And it was working.

Then came in the order for forty pounds. It was from a food truck owner named Chuey Fu's. The truck was adopting a "menu of the brave" theme for the upcoming Riot Fest (a music festival in Denver). In addition to rattlesnake and mountain oysters, the chef required crickets. The order was four times larger than anything McGill had ever filled. Fortunately, her other conference coup was meeting the head of Big Cricket Farms. BCF, based in Louisiana, is the country's largest insect operation. McGill admired BCF as a pioneer in the edible insect industry. Most notably, she admired the company for converting a well-established pet-food insect production facility to accommodate insects for human consumption ("food insects" require all manner of regulation; "feed insects"—bred for pet lizards—none). The move paid off, leading to more demand. Accordingly, the company's president hired McGill to be the western wholesale distributor of BCF's edible insect production line.

This position had numerous advantages for McGill. Most notably it addressed the problem of volume. As we've seen, McGill was getting orders from all over Denver, perhaps most promisingly from a gluten-free bakery that wanted to bake with cricket flour. The problem was, at only a year-old, Rocky Mountain Micro Ranch did not yet have the capacity to produce such volume. But now, as McGill explained, she was able to complement her supply with BCF sourced flour and whole insects. Not only that, but she was making a not-so-marginal profit of 35 percent on what she sold at wholesale. It was in this capacity that she successfully provided forty pounds of crickets for Chuey Fu. It was also in this capacity that she could finally imagine a real future for her insect business.

◯◯◯

During my September visit I also returned to McGill's can. The zoning snafu had sent her down the road, to another, somehow more rundown, vacant lot. This one was littered with rusting cars from the Eisenhower era. It abutted a shack of a convenience store catering to the local Hispanic community. Across the street was a windowless bunker called the "Stone Night Club."

The air outside the red can was mountain cool. The air inside the red can was tropical hot. The black tent in the red can steamed like a sauna. The grey containers, stuffed with egg cartons (from the Hispanic grocery) to increase surface area, practically wilted. And this was all as it should have been.

"Good, good, good," said McGill. "It's really warm in here." She fiddled with a black box equipped with a small silver antenna—supplied by Bitwater—that would send her a text alert if a dramatic change in humidity or temperature took place. After replacing a light inside the tent, scooping some toasty smelling grains into a tray, and re-soaking a sponge that watered the crickets, McGill looked to the floor, put her hands on her hips, and huffed in annoyance. "Ew. Escapees."

Her critters were proliferating and fattening—not dying. But they were also escaping, evidently through the seal between the mini-screens and the plastic bin. "Watch your step," she said to me, as she grabbed an empty grey container, took off its lid, and laid it on its side. She then began to fill the container with food, wet sponges, and stacks of egg cartons. "The trick," she said, zipping the black tent as we stepped out "is to make it so comfortable in there that they never want to leave." A week later she sent me an two-worded email with the subject line "escapees."

"It worked!"

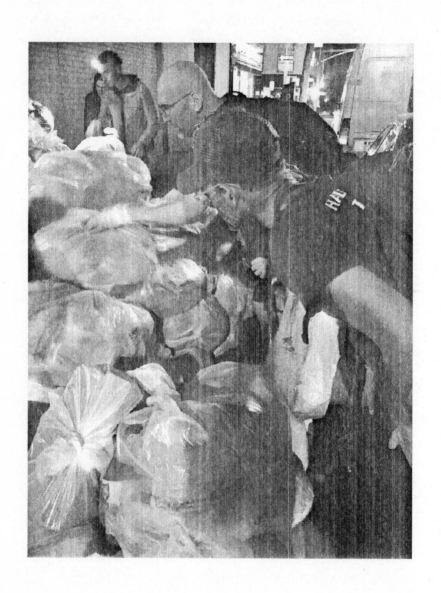

CHAPTER FOUR:

# The Tao of Trash

*"American cities are like badger holes, ringed with trash"*
—JOHN STEINBECK, *Travels with Charley*

On a cool June evening in Manhattan, I walked from Union Square to 16th St and 10th Avenue and climbed a flight of steps to the High Line—the borough's brilliant elevated public park. I was looking for a group of freegans whose Meet Up I'd arranged to attend. Freegan is a gimmicky word. But it makes its point. It blends "free" and "vegan" to describe a person who takes the vegan ethic to a more liberated and flexible extreme. A freegan is not a vegan. Nor is a freegan a bum. A freegan is a person who, driven by some serious level of disdain for consumer culture, works to reduce consumer waste by—in part—eating it.

The most common freegan pursuit, and the one that generates the most media attention, is an activity called dumpster diving. I was at the High Line in part because I wanted to learn more about the art of acquiring and, eventually, consuming edible trash. I also thought it might be worthwhile, in the effort to better understand food, to dive into a dumpster and reflect on the nature of my experience. Dumpster divers, after all, struck me as the ultimate culinary outliers. They presented themselves as more opportunistic but equally principled versions of Arthur Haines and the hunter-gatherers. The fact that the defining requirement of their diet was that the food they ate had been discarded—rather than be organic or local or meatless or paleo or whatever—suggested to me the kind of category-busting open-mindedness essential to the project of eating promiscuity.

Directions about where to find the group once I got to the High Line were vague. It's an expansive space and, with the weather being so nice, it was packed with people enjoying an evening outdoors. After wandering around and, through an odd sort of profiling, identifying citizens who appeared as if they'd be comfortable digging through garbage for dinner—and after interrupting two of the wrong groups, both of whom seemed mildly offended—I approached a tall, reed-thin man in his twenties, fairly confident in my instincts on this one..

He was wearing baggy linen pants, a tank top, and a flat drum over his shoulder. I asked him if he knew anything about a freegan Meet-Up at 16th and 10th. He did! In fact he, too, was looking for the group. "I'm Brett," he said, brushing sandy dreadlocks from his eyes and extending his hand. Brett and I walked around trying to locate the group's sponsor, Janet, who Brett thought he would recognize from previous freegan gatherings. As we poked into the more obscure corners of the High Line, Brett explained to me that he was only interested in finding fresh fruit on this evening's outing.

"Why?" I asked.

"Because that's all that I eat," he said.

We both spotted a small gathering of men and women sitting on layered rows of stone steps, slightly hidden from view. Brett waved to Janet and we went down to join the freegans. Janet, a school teacher from Brooklyn, welcomed us to the meeting and asked if we would introduce ourselves to the six attendees, suggesting that we say a word or two about our interest in learning about dumpster diving. Brett said that, for his part, he and his girlfriend had been eating a diet of exclusively fresh fruit for over four months. They saw no good reason to pay for apples and bananas if grocery stores were tossing apples and bananas into the trash. Plus, he added, he didn't have a job at the moment.

As Brett spoke, I got lost in my observations. Janet's clothes, as well as those of other attendees, seemed old. Like tired, worn down old. They looked to be sourced from a dumpster, or at least a Goodwill store. She

wore loose-fitting tie-dyed sweatpants, a threadbare t-shirt, and a faded
blue bandana to hold back a light tangle of brown hair. Later, as the wind
picked up, she added an ill-fitting red cardigan to the ensemble, in addition to fingerless gloves. As I made these sartorial notes, I wondered how
my heavily commercialized outerwear—Levi jeans, a Blackwing brand
t-shirt, a Camelbak backpack, North Face shoes, and a Patagonia ball
cap—must have looked to a gathering that, I was starting to sense, was
philosophically brand-averse.

Then suddenly everyone was looking at me to say something about
myself. I nervously explained that I was writing about people who, in
an effort to rethink the food system, went about acquiring their food in
ways that forced us to reimagine what it means to eat. People nodded.
There was some chatter. A woman said: "You chose well."

My initial interest in freeganism grew out of a college class I teach on
food ethics. A couple of my students had done some impromptu foraging through a few university cafeteria trash heaps and, impressed with
their scavenged items, upon which they saved considerable money, suggested that the topic might be worth exploring in a seminar discussion.
I agreed and circulated a video and a few articles on the topic. Twenty
honors students and I proceeded to have an engaging ninety-minute
conversation. After an excellent exchange of ideas (the liberal arts at
work), I walked away with what every good seminar discussion should
generate: a problem.

The problem, as I saw it, was this: did freeganism adequately address
the activity's underlying concern? When it came to food and freeganism, I was unsure about the logic behind cleaning up the food system's
waste by consuming it. Could the inner rationale of the dumpster dive—
in part, to fight against capitalism—backfire? Of course, as an activist
endeavor, dumpster diving unquestionably fit with at least one eco-eth-
ical touchstone of our time—the obligation to reduce food waste. Over
40 percent of food we produce in the United States is tossed in the trash.

Our cavalier treatment of trash represents a shameful mishandling of precious resources, not to mention an embarrassing testimony to our arrogant complacency with our bulging abundance. I have no doubts about the significance of reducing food waste. We need to do it and I appreciate how dumpster divers are addressing it.

But at this point food waste wasn't part of my problem with the freegans. My conundrum instead hinged on what they actually accomplish. When an ideologically informed group of activists rummages through capitalism's discard pile and, in many cases, driven by visceral hatred for the system, hauls home its excess, what is the result? Yes, they withhold their cash from the commercial behemoths they oppose, thereby voting with their dollars. And yes, I see the benefit in that withholding. But, at the same time, due to that same withholding, don't they indirectly help ameliorate the problem by reducing one of the system's most reputation-damaging problems: all that waste?

Perhaps I was outthinking myself on this one. But one of the most valuable functions of food waste as an official concern is to keep a constant black eye on the face of the food system. Could it be that scavengers, in so far as they envision a critical mass of roving freegan dumpster divers sopping up the juice on capitalism's plate, will leave the system looking cleaner than it is? Could freegans be helping the very entity they want to harm?

Despite this convoluted concern, I'd end up walking away with something better than an answer to the question I asked. Instead, I'd walk away with an answer to a question I didn't know to ask, an answer with much more powerful implications for the future of food.


## THE CODE OF THE CURB

Janet reviewed the meeting's agenda, which she had scrawled on a scrap of paper harvested from the sidewalk. After explaining that there would be a brief Freegan 101 primer, followed by an overview of dumpster diving etiquette and the logistics of our evening route, she asked if someone would please volunteer to be the meeting's "vibe watcher." Vibe watcher?

I'd never heard of a vibe watcher. But, as Janet explained, this was the person who monitored the meeting for signs that the mood was starting to become, as she put it, "hostile, tedious, or boring." Every member of the group, which had now grown to ten, looked around waiting for somebody else to be the vibe-watcher. No takers. "Well, I guess we can all do it," said Janet, undeterred by our apparent apathy. The vibes would be unwatched, at least by a designated watcher.

Janet's counterpart, a balding and bespectacled man in his fifties named David, agreed to share responsibility for the Freegan 101 presentation. He did so in part because his decades of experience qualified him to do so. But he also did so to dilute any appearance of hierarchy or undue dominance by a single individual. David's Meet Up profile mentioned his interest in fostering a sense of community and reducing his footprint on Mother Earth. His easy-going, affable manner seemed consistent with these qualities. As a person who isn't altogether comfortable in group situations, I couldn't help noticing what I often notice when I'm visiting a congregation of people: Everyone seemed to genuinely value being part of a community, thriving off each other's presence. This was a social as well as an ideological event, and David was kind of the friendly host.

Janet and David spoke about freeganism as primarily an ethic for which its signature act—dumpster diving—embodied its inner spirit. It wasn't an inner religious spirit so much as an inner secular spirit, an ethos rooted in communal self-sufficiency. And when it came to the dangers of boredom and tedium, these concerns were unfounded. Nothing anyone said about dumpster diving (which I was getting anxious to actually do) would in any way have required the officious intervention of a vibe watcher. Of course, if you happened to be a diehard proponent of Adam Smith, Milton Friedman, radical individualism, Ronald Reagan, or just a proponent of consumer freedom in general, woe to you. You would have quickly felt the vibe taunting your libertarian ethos. I had to laugh a little. Janet and Dave had a demeanor that would have made them perfect guests on an episode of *Mr. Rogers' Neighborhood*. But they were in fact ideological flame throwers as radical as anyone you could ever expect to meet (which, in a way, Fred Rogers was, too).

Freeganism espouses a fiercely anti-capitalist agenda. In its purest form, Janet and Dave explained, scraping and scavenging food served not only to feed people, but to affront the excesses of commercial capitalism while affirming the values of pared down communitarianism. "By bartering, salvaging, squatting, trainhopping, and dumpster diving," explained Janet, "you can avoid capitalist excess and share more goods with each other." This point was delivered in a voice that could have been reciting a phone number. No fists in the air tonight. Just action.

Another way to express this idea is to note that, by hoarding the dregs of the system, the truly free citizen could meet basic needs, distribute the surplus, and, in so doing, build organic communities around a pageantry of scavenged items, all the while keeping hard money out of the commercial nexus. Long time advocates such as Janet dedicated much of their non-working lives to putting these objectives into action. Rather than thunder away rhetorically at the excesses of consumer culture, they quietly took their thunder to the streets, using the system's waste to create a viable, if still largely imagined, alternative.

Nobody I spoke with claimed perfection when it came to the tao of trash. Occasionally even the most committed freegan became lazy and tapped into the system's undeniable convenience. Janet recalled an incident when, early in the summer, she purchased almond milk at a local grocery store. The next day, during a quick scavenge behind the same store, she found a case of discarded but fresh almond milk, one day past its expiration date. "The freegan gods will get you if are impatient," she warned.

When I asked if there was anyone in the group—our total had now grown to eighteen—who routinely scavenged for their entire diet, never buying food, not a single hand went up. But, as Janet and David were quick to affirm, there was a legendary local freegan couple—Gary and Nancy— who came as close as anyone knew to totally abandoning the retail grocery grid. They were scheduled to attend our meeting, but Janet guessed that they "were probably still scouting out the course for the evening."

By articulating freeganism in ideological terms, Janet and David were echoing freeganism's pseudo-official manifesto, an edgy if undisciplined sprawl of a document published in 2000 by one Warren Oakes, a man most commonly known for being the former drummer of the Florida-based punk band Against Me!28 In this broadside, Oakes delivers a litany of angry declarations: "working sucks," "you don't have to compromise yourself and your humanity to the evil demon of wage slavery," "by not consuming you are boycotting EVERYTHING," and "working to get money to buy things" is, above all else, a "waste of your life." The pamphlet reads like something written by a brooding high school Marxist with a flair for rhetoric. It's a characterization perhaps affirmed by the fact that, after publishing his screed against corporate capitalism, Oakes left his band and started up a burrito restaurant in south Florida.

But Janet and David are grown ups. They weren't terribly interested in adhering to the finer points of a high-octane manifesto. They were more intent to share the more reasonable acquisition strategies mentioned in Oakes's broadside. Foraging, bartering, "plate scraping," and home gardening—these were the pathways to revolution. Indeed, some members of the group, who were now regularly interrupting the presentation with advice gained from personal experience, actually had the temerity to approach strangers finishing a meal in a food court or large restaurant and ask if they wouldn't mind forking over the leftovers. "Saves a trip to the trash can," a French woman with stringy black hair visiting from Paris testified. Of course, the most common strategy of food acquisition—the one that we were here to learn about and, once the meeting ended, put into action—was dumpster diving.

The first thing to know about dumpster diving is that the act itself rarely involves a dumpster or diving. The term is more of a catchall phrase for rummaging through any form of trash in a quest for something salvageable and, preferably, edible. New York City, population 8.4 million, is the ideal locale for such an endeavor. In the city, if trash is placed curbside, or the dumpster sits on public property, then you, resourceful citizen of the metropolis, have a natural born right to transform that trash into treasure. Restaurants, of which there are roughly 24,000 in the five boroughs, are certainly ripe targets for a pick-up meal on the go. But if your interests hew to the long term—as in stocking the

28. http://freegan.info/what-is-a-freegan/freegan-philosophy/why-freegan-an-attack-on-consumption-in-defense-of-donuts/

larder, distributing goods to the homeless, or planning a dinner party—the curbs and dumpsters of grocery stores and markets (of which there almost 3500 in the city) are the smarter choice.

As Janet was clarifying this distinction, Gary and Nancy—the famous freegans—arrived. Both wore the same kind of patched-up, dead-to-fashion outfits as did Janet and Dave. The two carried plastic bags of food harvested from trash they'd scoured through on the way over. They immediately started sharing it with the group. Gary, who wore a well-trimmed Donegal beard and a Member's Only-type jacket, passed around packages of wasabi green pea crisps, only a couple of days past their date of expiration. Nancy handed out some protein bars marketed to women, also recently past due. She handed them to women.

Gary then asked if he could "have the floor" to present the evening's route. Janet and Dave ceded it to him. The plan, Gary explained, standing a little too imperiously on the top step, sort of like a General surveying his troops, was to hit three locations in the Chelsea area: Duane Reade, West Side Market, and Elm Health. Boom. Boom. Boom. He encouraged us to be disciplined in our maneuvers, as the city trash trucks, which worked on a tight schedule of their own, wouldn't wait for us to complete our search. Gary said that he was pretty sure all the managers at these venues were pro-freegan. A woman next to me wondered why all of Gary's metaphors were so martial. Nancy added that for those who preferred "organic" options, Elm Health, on 7th Avenue, would be well worth the wait.

Nancy made this comment without irony (truth be told, this was no crowd for irony). Still, it's hard not to see some humor in it. One would naturally think that, when it comes to eating trash, you'd be more or less content to get what you get. And this is mostly true—dumpster divers aren't prima donnas. They know they aren't ordering from a Nobu menu. But they also knew they had choices. Indeed, one of the first lessons I learned about rummaging through an urban trash heap is that the biggest challenge faced by freegans was the overwhelming abundance of what they harvested.

Both Dave and Janet told stories about struggling mightily to transport their scavenged fare by subway train. They resourcefully employed hiking backpacks, small grocery carts, and wagons rigged with siding to contain their load of treasure but, lacking cars, as most New Yorkers do, they were usually forced to leave behind considerable booty. Dave said that when he found more than he could carry he would usually "give it away on the spot, just share it with people on the street." Whatever the logistical response to the foraged abundance, it meant, as Nancy's remark intended, that even dumpster divers enjoyed a certain level of consumer choice.

It seemed fitting that the problem of abundance at the top end of the food chain was mirrored at the bottom. And indeed, the sheer volume of these dreg piles, all of it having trickled down from the highest peaks of the industrial food system, posed pressing health concerns for the itinerant freegans. As with the conventional shopper navigating the food section of Walmart, the freegan also had to monitor his choices in order to avoid the very same dietary challenges plaguing everyday consumers. The piles of waste freegans were sweeping into their rucksacks came from the very same system that had long trapped Americans such as the Reeds in the vice of too much.

Gary shared a story related to this point. He had recently found dozens of donuts from a small dumpster behind a Brooklyn bakery. His inner Freegan was thrilled with the cache of sweets; but the health-conscious consumer in him, not so much. His doctor had warned him to watch the carbs, so he wasn't planning to eat more than one or two. He knew he could easily offload the rest in the lobby of a nearby retirement home. But he also knew that the last thing most citizens living in that tower, many of them elderly and overweight, needed to do was spend their golden years feasting on free donuts donated by a guy who raided trash cans. Healthier food was harder to share, he conceded, because people were less interested in eating it. But when it came to junk food, "we find so much sweet stuff and people love it."

David agreed with Gary's assessment. He complained that the lemon pies he always found behind a Trader Joe's were irresistible—"that's how I got fat," he said, patting his gut. He called the chronic food quality concern the dumpster diver's "moral dilemma." It was, again, sort of sad, but the food system was so thoroughly corrupted with junk that even those eating from its trash heaps were, although to lesser degrees, suffering the ill effects of those eating from its apex.

Potential health consequences notwithstanding, the act of shifting through trash is not the free-for all you might expect. There are rules—comprising a strict code—that govern the chaos. As the scheduled ending time for the meeting approached, Janet reviewed the three most essential stipulations for socially responsible dumpster diving.

First, she advised, when a group of divers approached a site, it was imperative to make sure that other people in the area—mostly those with more obvious material needs—weren't denied first dibs at the stash. If a person was poking through a nearby trash can, a representative from the freegan team was obligated to approach that person and explain that they were preparing to legally rummage through a bunch of trash bags, that he was welcome to have the first shot, or could even join them in the plunder. Most freegans were also happy to forage on behalf of the homeless and those who seemed otherwise in need, if circumstances so warranted. Bottom line: be sensitive to those who might need that trash more than you did.

This rule highlighted to me the high level of social awareness that freegans brought to their work. To my knowledge there have been no demographic studies of dumpster divers. But it seems safe to assume (and this was certainly confirmed by my group) that they already enjoy access to basic resources (namely shelter and store-bought food) and in most cases much more than basic resources. One freegan Meet-up attendee, for example, was a graduate student at New York University. Another was on a student-abroad program from Norway. The woman from Paris was a filmmaker. Janet taught high school and Dave was a programmer.

It's morally essential to freegans that they do not deny free food to those who need it more than they do. And it's in the spirit of ensuring that access to scavenged food be as open as possible that freegan groups, including the New York City ones, routinely arrange tables of free food in public venues. Once a month, in order to foster group cohesion, the New York freegans also move the party inside, hosting potlucks of scavenged food at someone's apartment. The emphasis on sharing is consistent with the reality that, as we've seen, freegans almost always acquire more goods than they are able to consume. When I asked if this situation— offering access to people in greater need—was commonly acted upon, a seasoned member of the group told me: "much more than you'd imagine."

A second stipulation was designed to help shape the group's internal dynamics and communal identity. To prevent dumpster diving missions from devolving into competitive ventures driven by unfettered individualism (like what has happened with some yoga classes), but also to assure that those with special dietary preferences—in this case the vegan, gluten-free, and, well, fruitarian participants—were well attended to, the freegan ethic required that active participants vocally declare when they found something they thought worth keeping and, before packing it into their own backpacks, ask if anyone else wanted it (or some of it) first. For example, if you came upon a bunch of apples while digging through a bag of trash, you would be obliged to shout out: "Brett—I found a bunch of apples!" Brett, given his dietary preference, would then presumably have a fair chance to bring home a crisp sample of the only kind of food he ate. (This requirement—the shout out—would prove a little awkward/comical for me during our first stop at Duane Reade's, as we'll soon see.)

Janet and Dave were especially concerned about the third imperative—which has many parts: "Leave the site cleaner than when you found it, be polite to all citizens (even to those who said nasty things—which, as will also see, certainly happens), and do not under any circumstances hog the sidewalk." In other words: discipline. Do not, in your quest for righteousness, become blind to the world around you.

Many iconoclastic groups explicitly thumb their nose at societal conventions, especially the ones that they overtly oppose. They take pleasure in flaunting their departure from normality. Vegans can be that way. But freegans try to cultivate coolness under pressure. Although their behavior certainly antagonizes the status quo, often jarringly so, they are not interested in necessarily antagonizing the general populace, if for no other reason than they want people to join them. Nor are they even keen on drawing explicit attention to themselves. Still, as Janet did concede before we left the High Line, whenever a couple dozen people get together and rifle through trash bags on crowded city sidewalks, "you become something of a spectacle." No way around that, I suppose. But the underlying idea was simple and, in its way, quite charitable: Court the goodwill of the community and don't get in anyone's face. "We're just trying to highlight food waste and feed people," Janet reminded the assembled.

As the primer portion of the Meet Up came to an end, Janet requested a quick "meeting evaluation." Nobody doubted for a second that what she and Dave had shared was informative; everyone complimented them on their generosity and forthrightness. The only problem with the meeting, at least from the perspective of the visiting Parisian freegan filmmaker, was something that sounds pretty absurd but in fact proved to be charmingly emblematic of the freegan worldview: The steps on which we sat required some members of the community to sit above others. "Too much of a hierarchy," the French woman said.

As this point settled in, Brett proposed a unifying exercise, asking if the group would be open to impromptu "peace drumming" and, perhaps, chanting. Janet, keeper of the timepiece, demurred, saying that while she appreciated the idea, and understood that he was a talented peace drummer, if they didn't hit the street tonight's dinner would be picked up by garbage men and taken to a landfill. She shouted out one last bit of advice as we headed for the street: "Remember, nothing you find is off limits."

⌒○⌒

Tenth Avenue beneath the High Line shoots north like an arrow—unlike 11th Avenue, which kind of lolls lazily to the west. My team of freegans went straight up 10th at a brisk march until we reached 23rd St. There we made a hard right, moving in a tight peloton towards 8th Avenue,

where, on the curb outside Duane Reade's, stood dozens of bulging garbage bags, piled and folded on top of each other like a pack of seals on a
rock, just as Gary had promised.

"Dammit," one woman grumbled as she snapped on rubber gloves,
"*black bags*." Black bags meant more work. Specifically, we'd have to
open them before determining if what was inside was worth investigat-
ing. White bags were evidently transparent enough to save that step.
And not only did the black bags have to be unknotted, but the knots
themselves seemed to have been cinched by people with anger issues.
At least a dozen people converged on the heap and started wrestling
with the bags. There is, at this point, a funny picture of me. A line of
five freegans are bent over the trash in unison, fighting with the knots,
while I stood nervously in the middle of them, ramrod straight, like a
quarterback behind an offensive line before the play starts, unsure how
to proceed. Janet, who was on the other side of the pile, noticed my hesi-
tation and said, "It can be a big step to take food."

The group's collective effort to unknot every bag without ripping it
halted the chatter with a spell of concentration. And then, as if on cue,
bag upon bag came open, goods upon goods spilled into view, and a
more purposeful chatter resumed. "Candy!" was the first declaration I
heard. "Hard candy. Who wants it?" Immediately, someone yelled back,
"Why would you throw out hard candy?" but before he could finish a
young woman was almost screaming, "Mine! Mine! I need that! Please,"
and was scooping handfuls of it into her empty leather backpack.

She was thin and athletic looking, not the sort of person you'd really
suspect would gorge on lollipops. "You're going to eat all that?" I asked.
"No," she said, "I need it for an art project." I asked her what kind of
art she made. "Abstract," she said as she stuffed Jolly Ranchers into her
pocket. The call and response continued, highlighting the presence of
more hard candy, marshmallows, chips of all sorts, and granola bars.
Lots and lots of granola bars. Up until this point, I'd been standing to the
side, observing the chaos unfold, still playing the role of hesitant quarterback behind my steady offensive line. I'm not a squeamish person.
But something about the dive was keeping me at a distance. Perhaps it

was the parting comment a wry doctor friend of mine made when I left for New York: "Have a good time getting hepatitis!"

But eventually I screwed my courage to the sidewalk and found a slightly collapsed black bag, grabbed it roughly by the neck with my un-gloved hands (a sure sign of inexperience), cranked open the knot, looked inside its black maw, and yelled out my first official discovery as a New York City dumpster diver: "Condoms!" A virgin no longer, emboldened veteran that I now was, I rummaged even deeper, pushing aside Styrofoam packing material, and hollering with pride into the nighttime air the pragmatic object of my next find: "Tampons!"

I'd been warned. Still, it was hard for me to fathom just how much stuff there was for the taking. As my team picked through an industrial effusion of junk, the two problems we had discussed earlier became manifestly evident: space and time. This was a drug store, so there were more semi-durable goods (tampons, condoms, bottles of soda, boxes of cereal) than perishable fresh foods. The relative bulk of these items required the freegans, most of them hauling backpacks, to limit their catch, although some freegans would unpack, say, a box of cereal, take out the plastic bag containing the product, and leave behind the bulkier box. And as for time, Janet said we were running out of it, and quickly. She gave us seven minutes to retie and restack all the bags and do a thorough trash check of the sidewalk before moving to the next site. "Neater than we found it," insisted Dave, who was dragging away two small plastic bags of toiletries.

Just before leaving Duane Reade, I learned about a third problem that sometimes nagged the dumpster diver. As we were packing up, a woman announced with notable enthusiasm that she'd found soft bags of precooked wild rice. The discovery—finally!—of genuinely healthy food had considerable appeal after an hour of combing through a bunch of crap I'd never eat. Several of us went over to take a look, only to find that the store manager (presumably not freegan friendly), perhaps to dissuade the episodic mayhem of the dumpster dive, had sliced open the pouches holding the wild rice, making them far less attractive to consume. I took it as an obvious gesture of hostility—*don't come back here!*—and, now that I was sharing the field with my new comrades, all of whom I sensed to be goodhearted comrades, I found myself deeply annoyed with this small gesture to sabotage the sabotagers.

"Why do that?" I asked Janet. She shook her head and said that a surprising number of people did not like what we were out here doing. Public hostility to the collective dumpster dive effort became more obvious when we were digging through trash at the next site—the West Side Market (located at 7th Avenue and 15th St.) To get there, we flat out ran. Janet thought the trash trucks wouldn't give us more than thirty minutes at the site (she was wrong, they were late), and the load there was judged by Gary's recon mission to be substantial, maybe a third larger than at Duane Reade's, and full of fresh food. So we took off at a brisk pace. I wear a Garmin running watch and, out of curiosity, I set it to measure my pace. At one point I was running an 8:30/minute mile. Encountering piles of white bags (good!) and cardboard boxes (un-taped), we converged like the vultures we seemed intent on emulating.

By this point I had more than eased into the rhythm of the experience, seduced by the challenge, as well as the thrill of making especially bountiful discoveries. Running through the city on a beautiful evening, looking for free food, turned out to have an unexpected allure. I was flattered, moreover, when I undid a brown cardboard box to find a pile of greens—primarily arugula and spinach—and a roar of approval greeted my discovery. As I passed the box around, a well-dressed older man in his sixties walked over to us and, in a sharply angry tone, asked, "What do you think you're doing?" I looked over. "Are you *proud* of what you're doing? Are you homeless?" His voice was slurred, and he shuffled a little, recovered, and asked, "Can you justify this behavior?"

Such shit happens, of course. But this cranky codger with his shiny loafers, pressed slacks, and three-martini attitude was too much for me to bear. But Janet, with an almost eerie calm, went into grace-under-pressure mode. She repeated in the kindest voice possible her public service mantra: "We're just trying to highlight food waste and feed people." The man looked down on her as if she was a bug he wanted to squash. "You people," he seethed, "are drunk on your own privilege." He turned away and theatrically marched off. "You're just drunk," the guy next to me muttered as he sorted through the greens I'd found and put several handfuls in his saddle bag.

But the tide of curbside opinion soon turned. Five minutes later a young woman who had just moved into an apartment on the same block saw us in action and began asking how she could join us for the next outing. "You guys are awesome," she added. So there was that.

By this point, as we were cleaning up the sidewalk after our second surgical strike, I'd come to appreciate how, beyond dietary restrictions, different freegans had different standards about what they would take home and eat. One person I met, an Asian woman in her fifties, seemed completely undiscriminating. Whatever was technically digestible she took, presumably digested, and lived through the experience to become stronger. She sacked away in her feedbag piles of slimy greens, half-rotten apples, and even a package of browned-over ground beef with the plastic seal punctured.

I asked her if she felt safe eating food that had been so exposed and, in some cases, mildly decomposed (and, to be sure, it was *not* safe to do so). She seemed a little annoyed with my question, as if she was tired of people asking it. She sighed and explained that it was fine as long as you washed everything and cooked it well enough. "It has only been out here an hour or so," she noted.

Others adhered to more discerning standards. Several freegans I spoke to were happy to take food exposed to the elements as long as it looked and smelled fresh. Others, though, would only eat from nonperishable food sealed in containers. My own quickly evolving standard, to my surprise, proved to be on the more flexible end of the spectrum. By 10 pm, it had allowed me to eat, in addition to the wasabi crisps (from a bag), a bagel, two apples, some raw spinach, and a gulp of rice milk straight out of the container, all shared with the team. Worse meals have been consumed on the fly, for free.

By 11 pm, the city was in high gear. Sidewalks were crowded with people moving with to the hum of the street, the blab of the pave. In the middle of our third mission (at Elm Health), I took a break and texted a friend I'd planned on having dinner with (I'd been texting her all evening saying "a bit more time, sorry!"). In this text I suggested a rain check. But, she reminded me, this was New York and, she added, you could eat at midnight, and it was fun to do that. So no worries. She was happy to wait.

I dove into one last industrial plastic bag, sorted through boxes of "organic purple corn flakes," dinner rolls, and bananas. (Bananas!— Brett? Where's Brett? He'd already left.) So my last gesture before leaving was to thank Janet, hand to her a remarkably clean and perfectly ripened banana, and find a bathroom (Starbucks) to wash my hands. I then started walking toward the West Village, to meet my friend, who was waiting for me at a sushi place on University Ave. right near Washington Square Park.

My dumpster dive was an illuminating experience. The freegans I met were generous people who were morally concerned with the excesses of our food system, concerned enough to hunt down and swallow its waste, some of it borderline fetid. But, in part because of their generosity, they seemed, at first glance, to have very little to offer the food system of the future. By consuming the dregs of the very network they despised, they were, in a very modest way, cleaning it up. They did not, to any extent I could discern, push the food system in a new direction. They ostensibly did very little to challenge the actual form of the thing itself.

Still, even if I didn't fully embrace the ideology, I appreciated the movement's anti-capitalist stance. I understood its intention and could appreciate how it informed their actions. But the outcome of that ideology was something altogether different than what was articulated. Any prospect that freegan dollars being withheld from the grand culinary capitalist enterprise would somehow starve the beast from within struck me as implausible, especially given how few freegans were able to take their actions to the extreme place of a total boycott.

And then there was the problem of perception. The New York freegans were, to their credit, remarkably self-aware about how they were perceived. They worked hard to counter the notion that dumpster diving was crassly self-serving or little more than hipster slumming (as suggested by the drunk guy who verbally accosted us). The perception is hardly the fault of the freegan, who, again, seemed to do everything possible to be unassuming, decent, and polite. But there is evidently something inherent in the idea of trash—maybe our evolutionary association of it with disgust—that seemed to make it impossible for a lot of observers to accept as food. So, for the moment at least, my skepticism seemed to be in the same place as it was before I went dumpster diving.

But that changed when I got downtown.

I arrived at the West Village sushi place by 11:30. Within minutes of entering the restaurant, my friend and I, menus in hand, were sitting at the bar interpreting a multi-page oceanic underworld of consumer choice. Tuna, snapper, clams, sea urchin, salmon, eel, bonito, toro,—the list was long and, yes, diverse, and most of the goods were displayed right in front of us, jammed into plastic cases, much of flown in that day from around the world.

But this was totally the wrong kind of list, the wrong kind of diverse. This food should not have been slabs of pink, red, and white flesh pressed into the shield in front of us; it should have been flesh on the bodies of fish swimming in the sea. All of this food was high impact, a further drag on the oceanic ecosystem, where most fish are overfished, shipped in from netherworlds by airplane, and, alas, thrown out. I refrained from ordering fish, sticking instead to vegetable sushi, steamed edamame, spring rolls, and a beer. The chef gave me a look. My friend had a little sashimi but otherwise ordered more or less as I did. Still, the bill came to $150.

Not a shocking figure, especially in New York City. But not totally unworthy of reflection either. It's not a question I typically ask on the rare occasions when I dine out, but then again I'm typically not dining out after an evening spent rummaging through trash. So I found myself wondering: What exactly was I paying for? The answer, revealing itself on long post-dinner walk back to my midtown hotel, and then requiring an hour of note taking, turned out to be more complicated than I'd imagine. But the short answer was that I paying less for "food" and more for "the experience of eating." And it was in my realization of this distinction that the wisdom of the dumpster dive finally bloomed into something more significant than a quixotic idea about overturning capitalism or, less quixotically, making a dent in something as tangible as food waste. It was in that distinction that I began to take seriously the proposition that the restaurant as we know it may also need to be fundamentally reimagined as an element of the future food system.

Dumpster diving may do nothing to confront capitalism. But it fosters a dramatically pared down and unadorned way of looking at food. From the perspective of the street, a carrot is a carrot; an avocado is an avocado; soybeans are soybeans; rice is rice; beer is beer. You find it; you share it or keep it; you consume it; you move on, nourished and sated. But in the context of an architecturally sleek sushi place in a fashionable part of Manhattan, under the curatorial care of an enrobed sushi chef wielding cutlery that costs more than monthly rent, in a dining room of coupled-off diners secluded from each other, the meaning of these ingredients becomes transformed into something altogether more complicated. And not necessarily in a good way.

Restaurants—like the food system—have their own elaborate chain of events that usher us into a "food experience." The events that comprise this experience—the airlifted fish, the attractive hostess, the abstract art hanging on the walls, the dim lighting, the polished server on site "to take care" of patrons, and so on—have a way of alienating higher-end restaurant food from the food itself (of course, middlebrow chain restaurants do the same but in a very different way). Consider the elaborate menu descriptions—"Kent garden pea puree"—frequently reducing food to senseless verbiage, and the distance only increases. Calorically and nutritionally what we eat remains the same, but its essence as food for sustenance or nourishment yields to food as culture, luxury experience, literary puffery, and entertainment, not to mention a $150 check.

It's sometimes said that all food "comes with a story." Dumpster diving has a nice way of getting to the simplest version of the narrative. A conventional restaurant, by contrast, draws it out into something episodic and indulgent.

The translation from "food as food" to "food as experience" or "food as story" is something we widely celebrate as defining historical and cultural developments . It seems the foodie media cultivates heroic narratives woven around cuisine and those who prepare it as form of highbrow nostalgia. It's one of those assumptions—the experience of formally eating out—that we practically never question. Which is strange because, just as with agriculture per se, eating out is a relatively new behavior as well. Beyond all the marketing jargon and foodie-hype, there are some unsavory ulterior motives that we might do well to appreciate. Notably, perhaps more than ever, high-end dining might be all about the rarest and finest talent, ingredients, and taste (with Chez Panisse as the model). But, as a result, it also offers a cheap means of achieving status, distinction, and, for the fancier venues, bragging rights.

And while there's always a case to made for the pursuit of status, distinction, and bragging rights through culinary consumption, the freegans remind us that "food as experience" has social consequences that I can assure you most food writers will never notice, much less reveal. Through their gritty egalitarian ethos, the freegans remind us that eating is more than a social act—it is, when made exclusive, a social act with consequences. They remind us that, for one, when you spend a lot of money in a restaurant, it's not just food that's alienated from food. Nor is it just people alienated from food (no matter how tasty the food is, as taste is perhaps the most superficial way to connect with food). *People are alienated from people.*

Restaurants channel us into culinary classes. They use food to make us strangers to each other. They segregate us by the varied experience of our plates. Like shoes and vacation spots, restaurant experiences drive hard wedges into society. They turn food into weapons of the wealthy, promoting the narcissism of big differences. Privileged consumers have made Facebook postings of fancy food a cottage industry that aims to price out the masses. The dining hoi polloi eat Sysco-delivered food microwaved in the "kitchen" at Applebees and typically do not text their friends pictures of their fried cheese sticks and margarita mixed drink (well maybe they do but what that means is for another rant). If you don't think this distinction drives us apart, then you must think that nothing drives us apart.

As you might guess, I generally dislike eating out. I especially dislike eating out at fancy places (I sound like a lot fun, right?). But I say this after having done it a lot, often with some serious gusto, most of it back in my twenties and early thirties, when I made it a conspicuous mission in my life to eat at Europe's and America's best restaurants. I don't even want to think about the grand sum of money and time and utter foolishness I dumped into eating all that rich, fine, absurdly fine food. Naturally, I can now look back and ask myself the obvious questions: Did I consume absolutely stunning food? Did I enjoy tastes that made me swoon? Did I sit in gorgeous rooms full of gorgeous people? Did I eat foie gras at a café in Paris that made my eyes water with pleasure?

*You bet I did.*

But I was immature and insecure and used food as a social booster into a world I ultimately found to be shallow, incurious, indulgent, and, really, not the least interested in knowing where food truly came from. Worse, however unknowingly, I was contributing to systematic food waste, chronic worker exploitation, tremendous greenhouse-gas emissions, and the polarization of the food system along exclusionary lines that my new freegan friends—who were doing their best to rectify some of these problems—rightly found abhorrent. The more I thought about it, especially in the context of the freegan experience, the more I agreed with these fearless trash pickers. Garbage is the ultimate leveler.

Imagine a world without traditional restaurants. No more ridiculous faux literary descriptions of otherwise honest food ("scratch cooked," "house-made," "agri-doux," and my favorite, "hand-cracked eggs"). No more clichéd restaurant reviews (with all those "decadent" deserts, "cozy" interiors, "yummy" food all "washed down with" some vintage or other), no more waiting a month to score a 5 pm reservation at the latest faddish place, with names like "Barley Swine," "Sway," and "Wink," spending a couple of hundred dollars, shooting an Instagram food story, and forgetting what you ate a day later. No more chain imitations that adopt the ersatz trappings of superior eateries—all those Olive Gardens and Outback Steakhouses, Appleby's and Chili's. And best of all: no more fast food.

"But what about jobs" goes the familiar refrain. As for the culinary talent that would be forced from the kitchens of America's restaurants, they could take it to the streets. Food trucks, open-air food courts, family style food halls all lend themselves to less waste, greater flexibility, more simplicity, community cohesion, and easier, more democratic access. No entrée over ten dollars, if I were king. Craft beer everywhere. This is what I learned from the freegans. And I'm aware that it sounds a little nuts. But I look at it this way: If a new restaurant in a Bobo section of Austin, my town, can convince people to spend $22 on a hamburger (which I assure you it can), then I'm convinced some innovative young chef with a renegade flair could get these same people *not* to spend $22 on a hamburger. He could, instead, sell something more original, just as tasty, and far more sustainable. From the helm of a humble food truck, he could convince them to eat promiscuously at an affordable cost. And he could, in the end, invest the choice with real meaning—meaning that's more about substance than style, more about food than the experience of food.

There are other ways to enjoy real food than going to a trendy restaurant, segregating ourselves (on so many levels) from others, paying too much for the "dining experience," participating in the myth-making of fancy food, wasting even more food than we do at home, and moving further and further away from the actual food itself, not to mention what it means to eat it. There are better ways to co-exist with food, not to mention each other.

We don't have to start eating out of trash bags to achieve this goal. But in doing so, my dumpster divers introduced me to a tao of trash that, while not necessarily uprooting capitalism from its foundation, reminds us that food is, for all the distractions we place between ourselves and what we eat, ultimately about physical sustenance. Dress it up in culture, history, lore, myth, and legend, food is just food. The freeegans, the weirdos, the outliers, the rebels—all of them show that the essence of food can be honored with an approach to eating that stresses fellowship, political idealism, community values, and, every now and then, a delicious burst of streetside flavor. Again, when you are eating free meals from trash heaps, everyone is at the same table. It is for this realization, more than any other, that I thank the freegans for what they taught me about food and what it could be.

♡○○

The next morning, after only a few hours of sleep, I had to catch a train out of the city. After rushing on foot to Penn Station, only to find that my train was delayed by an hour, I walked back outside to look for a bagel shop I recalled being on the other side of Madison Square Garden. I turned the corner onto 33rd and spotted a black lattice trashcan stuffed with white paper bags full of large pretzels. Tentatively, greedily, I paused and looked around. Then I approached the can. Several construction workers were eyeing me, gauging my next move, observing me contemplate this overflow of edible debris. For the second time in less than twelve hours, I screwed up my courage and grabbed two pretzels. I stood at the can and bit into one—a fat, salt-encrusted twist of dough—and moved on.

I finished the first salty pretzel as I walked back to the station. Down in the waiting area, I decided to adorn the next pretzel with purloined condiments. I grabbed a napkin, helped myself to a packet of catsup and a packet of mustard from a deli, sat on the ground under the schedule board next to the exit steps, gave the second pretzel another once-over, squirted my condiments on it, and ate that one, too. And there it was: my first freegan breakfast—two fat pretzels. Way too many carbs. But cheap and, for better or worse, unforgettable.

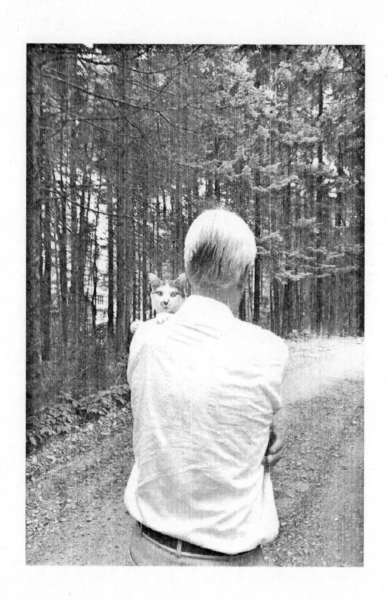

# CHAPTER FIVE:

# Underwater Treasures

*"There are heroes in the seaweed."—Leonard Cohen*

## LARCH'S LARK

People who live by the sea usually have an origin story. For Larch Hanson, a tall, handsome, sinewy man in his early seventies, it began in Minnesota and, after an impromptu jag through central Florida, continued into far northern Maine, where he still lives with his wife, Nina. The year was 1965 and the chosen mode of transport was a BMW motorcycle. Larch skidded to an end on a wooded patch of land that jutted into an isolated bay. The trip ended, he told me, "because it ended."

Larch was so enchanted that, with money borrowed from his father—a Minnesota farmer and an extension agent—he bought the land where his trip ended, all seven acres of it. He has since built a sprawling clapboard home (in my notes I called it "an elaborate cabin with a turret"), ringing it with at least a dozen elevated planks buried in the woods and topped with expensive, sturdy tents for guests. What he said of the invasive green crabs that now choked the cove at the edge of his property, he also said of his arrival in Maine: "I was here for good." And he was. Larch really doesn't travel. People travel to Larch.

Larch's land is isolated and charming. It stretches along the Maine coast, on the edge of a town called Steuben. The land is also gorgeous and rare, a pristine example of a New England forest growing to the edge of the cold Atlantic without the barrier of a sandy beach. This geological quirk, in addition to the place's relative inaccessibility, helps contain tourists in the touristy places, leaving Steuben for the locals to live free or die in[29] (which, in one case, meant letting a Confederate Flag of someone's angry disposition fly high above a ramshackle squat of a trailer I spotted on the drive in). Acadia National Park is an hour to the southwest. But the 2,500,000 annual visitors to that postcard-perfect plot of paradise have little idea or inclination to seek the grittier shoreline of Steuben.

On an unseasonably warm weekend in August, I made the journey and, after a short run in Acadia National Park, went to see Larch. When I arrived, after getting badly lost, a young woman was sitting on a log in the wooded parking area. I introduced myself. "Yeah, hi he's expecting you," she said. "Just go in and walk around till you find him." I found Larch upstairs in his office. He led me back outside and we meandered around the house, chatted, and then we headed down to the cove with his cat, who followed us with the loyal perseverance of a dog. Soon we were standing in a thick copse of maples and white pines, looking out into a body of water called Gouldsboro Bay. I could hear the trees around us creaking in the warm wind. A hawk sailed from one branch to another. Every time I asked specific questions, Larch would steer them back to the topic of reincarnation, which, as a practitioner of Tibetan Buddhism, he believed in.

Larch, who now held his cat on his shoulder as if burping an infant, pointed to two small grey dots sitting in the low-tide muck. He grew a little somber, wistfully identifying them as his trusted skiffs. For the last thirty-eight years, he told me, he has used those little boats, which he also built with his own hands (out of red cedar), to ply his trade. One motored him to sea (single outboard engine), and the other, which he tugged behind him, held his catch.

"I'm Larch Hanson," he declared. "The seaweed man."

---

29. Of course, this is the slogan of New Hampshire, but you get the idea.

Initially, the idea of a seaweed harvester—much less a seaweed harvester who believed in reincarnation—sort of made me laugh. I kept thinking of that old *Saturday Night Live* skit where John Malkovich plays "Len Tukwilla," a "driftwood artist" from the Pacific Northwest who takes the art world by storm. Len gathers wood, decorates it, ponders it, muses over it, and then, dreamily, elevates the wood into art and himself into an artiste. Hanson, too, gathers seaweed, does a lot of contemplative musing, indulges in an occasional bout of self-elevation, and calls the whole arrangement not so much a living as a life.

As I'd quickly learn, though, Larch's work, in contrast to Tukwilla (that melancholic slacker), is a testament to vigorous physicality. There's a reason Hanson has the raw-boned build of a wide receiver. His job— which he calls "good body work"—demands a convergence of physical engagement, most notably some herculean balance of finesse, strength, patience, and the willingness to take on forces that would conquer most men half his age—elemental powers like, you know, the ocean and the wind. There's not much that's conventional about Larch Hanson. But he did evoke for me the stereotype of the stubborn old Yankee who refused to be cowed by external circumstance, leaning into forces primal and unforgiving with dogged fortitude.

Hanson harvests seaweed within a five-mile radius of his house. He's never ventured beyond. "That's my rowing distance," he told me. "If my motor goes out, I can go home; I don't go beyond what I can row." Depending on the location and type of the particular seaweed species he's harvesting, he will sometimes leave shore as early as 2 am, arrive at his chosen location an hour later, and spend two more hours hauling over a thousand pounds of kelp from the ocean floor into his oaken skiff. He'll then head back in time for breakfast, which Nina, his wife, makes for him.

His early departure time primarily has to do with tides. But another reason for the early departure is to get to the seaweed blooms before the commercial guys do. "It's a derby out there," says Larch (more on the competition soon). But another part of the idea is to be done with work early in the day. "I've got so much else I want to do," he said. He was referring to the infrastructure of a commune/retreat center that he's building in the woods behind his home. There are also many upkeep tasks relating to his drying barns, which line the outside of his house like a row of barracks.

If Hanson is busy, he doesn't rush. On the wall of one of his seaweed drying rooms he has written the words "quietude and stillness." When he's alone at sea, he appreciates the silence and values being "embedded in the wholeness" of such stillness. His middle of the night walk to the black shoreline is about a quarter mile through a patch of forest. He can—and sometimes does—do it with his eyes closed. He reminded me that he was born on October 13, "the day of the survivor." He told me he has experienced only one instance of true oceanic fear. A storm brewed up from nowhere, forcing him to an unfamiliar shore. He turned over his boat, crawled beneath it, and took a nap.

"I have night vision," he told me. Indeed, at sea, he rarely uses artificial light. When he senses that it might be an opportune moment to blow a foghorn, such as when he hears another ship plowing his way, he bellows into the ink dark air a guttural "HO!!!!! HO!!!!!!!" He told me this in a quiet voice, almost whispering the words.

When I asked him to demonstrate an actual HO! HO! we were sitting in his large, cedar-lined home office. He demurred. "It would scare my neighbor," he said, "and she just moved in." This struck me as strange, given that that the only apparent neighbor lived in a house far down the dirt road, on the way to the cove, at least a quarter mile away.

After situating me in front of his computer to look at some gorgeous seaweed pictures taken by his wife, Larch waited until I was distracted by the slide show, a little off my guard, and then he hollered out a full throated "HO!!!!! HO!!!" I think the rafters rattled. I nearly fell out of my chair. I'd only known this guy for about an hour. But here he was, this silver-haired survivor, playing a joke on me.

"Loud, right?" he said, his torso shaking with muted laughter.

"Hope your neighbor's okay," I said.

## TAMAR AND KEVIN LEAVE THE CITY FOR THE FARM

Down the rock-rimmed New England coast, in Barnstable, Massachu-setts, situated on the northern part of Cape Cod, Tamar Haspel and Kevin Flaherty told a different how-I-got-to-the-ocean narrative. They did so as we sat in their living room overlooking a staid and sparkling inland pond. The house so closely borders the water I could not, from my vantage point in a chair (with a computer attached to its left arm) see the shoreline. I only saw sliding doors, a small deck with a smoker on it, and then a shimmering expanse of black water.

Tamar and Kevin, married and in their fifties, came to Barnstable from Manhattan in 2009. Kevin, with greyish hair pulled into a firm pony-tail, worked for decades on the trading floor of the city's stock exchange. Tamar is lanky and boney with a short, boyish thatch of brown-gray hair and expressive hazel eyes. She wrote (and still writes) freelance articles on the food industry. Her writing gigs would eventually culminate in a food column for the *Washington Post*, where her articles now garner (deserv-edly) accolades of the James Beard Award variety.

Saturated with the exciting pulse and pace of New York, and then eventually enervated by it, the couple decided to seek quieter ground in a place where they could, as one might, experiment with self-sufficiency. More space was needed. Tamar wanted chickens. She also wanted a gar-den, easier access to deer hunting and fishing, as well as the opportu-nity to test her untested quest for autonomy. Kevin wanted these things, too. He also wanted the chance to pursue his ongoing interest in finance (which he eventually would like to teach) in a more personal and less hectic setting than New York City.

Barnstable, where 50,000 people live on seventy-two square miles, is about 102 times less dense than the island of Manhattan. It seemed the right spot—the couple has about two acres of land—to breathe deep, reboot, and, if not go off the grid, at least tiptoe around it. It was a place, as Tamar explained, where she and Kevin could "try to stay connected to the idea that food has to come from somewhere."[30]

My own journey to the Cape, where I had only been once before,

---

30. http://starvingofftheland.com/contact-information-2/

started from Larch's wayward compound. I made the trip in a rental car that vibrated like an old washing machine when it hit 60 mph. Worse, it was about a seven-hour drive, a time that, with my central Texas sense of distance, I didn't think quite possible in quaint New England. I broke up the trek with a stop in Portland, Maine, where I ate dinner—which, as it so happened, included a pile of stringy seaweed—at a Whole Foods market. I motored on as the sun set and stayed the night in Gloucester, Massachusetts, a global fishing center north of Boston, where I ate at a delicious tofu/dill sandwich at a crunchy-hippie-bobo grocery called the Common Crow. A tofu sandwich in the country's most iconic fishing village? Call it a lone moment of quiet, outlier-inspired, promiscuity.

Early the next morning, well before the sun rose, I walked to Gloucester's commercial port and witnessed the tail end of the global aquatic food chain surge towards its destination. Fishermen loaded their catch into the auction warehouse, auctioneers propositioned buyers with their staccato of commercial verse, distributors loaded trays of iced snapper into Legal Sea Foods trucks, and the diesel lories hauled forth the catch to the metropolis, leaving in their wake the rancid odor of an especially hellish landfill. Just one short moment in the food chain, but one that diners ordering fresh fish that night in Boston would never be asked to consider.

From Gloucester I made the two-hour trip to Barnstable, dutifully following Tamar's non-Google-Map instructions. They ended with "you'll see our shack at the end of the long gravel driveway" and "don't be late." I made absolutely sure to adhere to this advice. I got there early, parked "downtown," and walked around. The air, in contrast to Gloucester, smelled of salt and lavender. Then, after having a cup of coffee in a tiny café, I drove to the designated address. Tamar was correct about her place—it had shack status. There was an outdoor shower, a rusty truck, and debris scattered in the yard. But, still, it was more chic shack than cracker cottage. The mess struck me as perhaps a little cultivated.

As life progressed for Tamar and Kevin, they would not, as reality (winter) set in, become full-fledged, self-sufficient back-to-the-landers. This outcome, realized mercifully early on into their leave-the-city time-line, was confirmed by the revised title of Tamar's active blog: "Not Living off the Land." "At the most," she explained, "we could provide 30 percent of what we ate—and even that took a ton of work." She looked fiercely at me when she said this, as if it was somehow my fault. Kevin, for his part, never found his footing in the constricted world of Barnstable finance. That particular pond was smaller than he had anticipated. "You can't fight John Henry," he said.

But you can grow oysters. The couple carved out what would prove to be a more suitable, if unexpected, niche, one that they could pursue together. Drawing on a mixture of gumption and Google, they acquired a two-acre lease of Barnstable Harbor's sea floor and, with the additional help of YouTube, taught themselves—and are still teaching themselves—how to be oyster farmers. Neither Kevin nor Tamar would ever have guessed they'd end up doing such work. They had no prior experience with mollusks whatsoever (with the notable exception of eating them). But—led by Kevin, whom I sensed had a knack for diving into unfamiliar projects with the intensity of a hedgehog—they assumed the task with the enviable attitude that, if others could do it, well then, so could they. This DIY spirit was something I saw a lot of in the course of my research. It left me deeply reassured. Not just in the confident and ongoing spark of human ingenuity, but also in the permission it offered us to think about starting over when it comes to food.

About being on time: Barnstable Oysters was a company whose existence ultimately came down to one overriding, time-sensitive, and beautifully mysterious phenomenon: tidal shifts. "The moving tides are what they are," wrote Rachel Carson in *The Sea Around Us*. For Tamar and Kevin, they were—or at least had become—everything. The couple consulted tide charts the way the rest of us consult watches (or, I guess, phones). Between high and low tides, fourteen feet of Atlantic seawater—an unusually generous flow—surged in and out of the harbor. These magnetically monitored motions washed Tamar and Kevin's oyster beds—their "farm"—in a daily soup of nutrients, plumping them into salty sweetness. It would be like a land-based farmer getting the exact same amount of rain every day, a blessing of a delivery that enabled him to predict the exact tumescence of his corn kernels.

Threading the needle of the tides, which Tamar and Kevin agreed to do with me, required more than my timely arrival. It also required that, once out on the farm, the work be efficient. At the end of the day, my punctuality, as well my modest efforts on the farm and in the kitchen, mild as they were, would certainly offer rewards to reap.


## THE DYING DEEP BLUE SEA: ECOLOGY

The stories that follow about Larch, Kevin, and Tamar are oriented around marine life. More so, they're about the future of marine life, which is, by many measures, the bleakest aspect of an already bleak food system. Larch, Kevin, and Tamar make their living by extracting animals and plants from the sea. How they do so is interesting. We'll get to those details. But what's just as significant is how they *do not* do so. How they *refuse* to do so. This distinction matters a great deal. It's one of the essential pivots to a future food system that is, to use again an overused word, sustainable. What they do not do allows these producers to cut the prohibitive anchors of the past and pursue food-based diversity through models of production that improve the aquatic environment and reduce harm to animals. Rather than accept unsustainably extractive methods as normal, people such as Larch, Tamar, and Kevin preserve and even enhance the deep blue sea's life-sustaining resources.

This is nothing personal against the hardworking fishermen of Gloucester, Massachusetts. But responsible oyster and seaweed farming, unlike unfettered fishing and fish farming, make the ocean viable and diverse, establishing the basis for recovery, rather than depleting it with relentlessly short-term calculations made to satisfy bottom-line operations such as Legal Sea Foods. If the Gloucester fisheries would leave the oceans to the likes of Larch, Kevin, and Tamar, while sending their fishermen into more responsible lines of work (breweries?), and if consumers would adjust their tastes accordingly, the ocean would become the most promiscuous and planet-healing force on earth. And consumers would be healthier and better satiated as a result.

Fish typically get overlooked in today's food discussions. Mainstream talk about protein sources focuses on land animals—the kind that we've seen cause severe ecological damage. But the number of finfish we kill for food is at least five times the number of chickens we harvest annually. And the environmental devastation that ensues is decidedly worse. A majority of fish is wild caught. The outcome of this extraction is mass endangerment and extinction. The rest of our fish is farmed—which also leads to endangerment and extinction (primarily because the feed for farmed fish comes from wild fish). Ecologically speaking, then, the farmed/wild debate is generally moot. Both contribute to an absolute ecological mess.

What's further worrisome in terms of sustainability is how rapidly rates of fish consumption are on the rise. In the 1960s, per capita fish consumption was a modest 9.9 kg. In 2013 in was 19.7 kg. Nothing indicates that it will slow down anytime soon. By 2050, rates are expected to have risen by another 82 percent. What's now happening on the high seas, whether on farms or on fishing vessels, to sustain this rising demand is nothing short of environmental piracy. Global fishing vessels rob us of a healthy and accessible aquatic future. They perpetuate an unregulated plunder of oceanic resources that, again, will benefit the few at the expense of the many.

They do this not because they are horrible people or cruel corporations. They do it because that's what consumers want; that's what we consider normal. They do it to fuel our eating habits that, again, seem to require the most inefficient expenditure of resources to sustain diets that are increasingly homogenous and unhealthy. A mere ten kinds of fish comprise 90 percent of the seafood we eat (by volume).[31] But it's not just ten types of fisheries that are in danger of collapsing. Due to the scope and depth of international fishing ventures, the world's oceans are, as a whole, experiencing what the Pew Oceans Commissions calls "a silent collapse."

The only reason it's silent is that we're not listening. And we're not listening because fish live where we can't see them, the industry is off shore, and the products are considered to be healthy. While most fish is certainly better for us than the insane amounts of land animals we eat, there is nothing healthy about oceans purloined of their biodiversity. If

---

31. http://www.progressivegrocer.com/industry-news-trends/regional-supermarket-chains/10-most-popular-fish-make-90-volume

the dangers don't come from inside our bodies, they'll just as assuredly come from without. One way or another, our addiction to fish makes us vulnerable.

To appreciate the dangerously aggressive nature of this decline in marine biodiversity, consider the case of salmon. Tasty, healthy, versatile (and, for some reason, a food we prefer dyed pink) salmon has become a staple across the social spectrum of the American menu (well, it hasn't trickled down to fast food yet). One seafood distributor praises our "soaring appetite for the product."[32] But salmon, before becoming exclusively a "product," once thronged the Pacific Northwest. Hell, salmon once thronged the waterways of New England. It was, at one time, endlessly available.

Today, over half of the 400 salmon stocks are at risk of extinction. One hundred and six have already become extinct. [33] In 2015, salmon fisheries experienced their "worst ever" shock to the system when 1.2 million sockeye salmon were predicted to return to spawning grounds and (without sending word why) never did. The head of the First Nations Wild Salmon Alliance concluded with the understatement that, "salmon stocks are in grave danger." This trend is no anomaly. In fact it's the ultimate norm for nearly all species of marine fish. What's happening to salmon is little more than a microcosm for what's happening with oceanic fish worldwide. The combination of fishing technology and fishing methods—designed to meet exploding consumer demand—best illuminates the nature of the devastation.

Most fish are caught with nets, some of them as large as a football field. Trawl nets, gill nets, seine nets—whatever the precise weapon—drag the bottom of the ocean and scoop fish from the sea without discrimination. Everything caught in this weighted and undiscerning rake gets cranked to the surface by the kind of crane used to build skyscrapers. The massive catch is then cinched into a wrecking-ball of wriggling flesh, and dropped on deck to be sorted by seasonal workers paid poorly to do some of the most horrible and dangerous work on earth.

---

32. http://academy.pittmanseafoods.com/en/2015/05/no-slowdown-in-the-growing-popularity-of-atlantic-salmon/
33. Kemmerer, 60

What falls on deck is an obvious hodgepodge. It includes animals caught unintentionally, a lot of them endangered mammals such as seals, sea lions walruses, and dolphin, the last of which 6 million have been killed since the introduction of tuna nets in the 1950s. About 40 percent of fish that are taken from the ocean are unwanted by the fishing vessels. They could take it or leave it. So they leave it. About 90 percent of it dies. The market—which, as we've seen, prefers only about ten types of fish, determines what gets turned into product. The rest gets tossed back into the big drink as "bycatch."

Big fish—top of the food chain species—are frequent examples of such wasted aquatic life. Ninety percent of large predatory fish have been fished to the point of collapse. The removal of these predators creates ecological havoc. In some cases, fish under pressure to replace their declining numbers have gone into micro-evolutionary overdrive toward early maturation. To reproduce earlier is, evolution has determined, one way to stay ahead of the nets. But, the evolutionary response, as old as life itself, is still no match for the trawls that scrape the ocean floor.

Today, overall, some 63 percent of all fish species are overfished. Some scientists have therefore concluded that, due to fishing technology and methods, by 2048, "all commercial fish and seafood species will collapse."

## THE DYING DEEP BLUE SEA: ETHICS

Further complicating the sad case of fish is recent research showing that our scaly underwater brethren may be smart, feeling creatures, every bit as sentient as the farmed land animals we eat. This is, I admit, a tough pill to swallow. I almost hesitate to draw attention to the issue because its implications (I mean, if you care) are so drastic it almost encourages a "screw it all" response. But still, when considered in light of the truly hopeless ecological situation perpetuated by global fisheries, all to feed consumers a narrow range of food, this research might further help us get beyond the whole idea of eating fish as integral to human existence, clearing more space for unsung heroes in the seaweed.

In terms of documenting basic fish intelligence, researchers have made critical discoveries. We now know that fish exhibit advanced Pavlovian responses to food offerings, a behavior that highlights "associative learning" rather than simple expressions of instinct. In one study, fish placed in a new environment reliably recalled where and at what time they were fed. They memorized this information after only fourteen trials (as opposed to forty for rats, whom we know to be pretty smart).

Relatedly, fish have demonstrated a navigational ability that outstrips that of human toddlers. When introduced to novel settings, they quickly associated safe regions (stable rock pools) with immobile geographical features (such as a patch of grass). When tides were suddenly manipulated, they sought out those pools, thereby avoiding being beached on a sandbar during an unanticipated disturbance.

Other findings edge us closer to thinking about fish as conscious decision-makers. Young salmon have been shown to imitate their elders in social situations. When presented with a new food in captivity, they will hesitate before cautiously testing the food. But when they are housed in a tank with older fish, and when they witness these elders eating the strange food, they follow the example, chomping away with far greater aggression and, it seems, confidence.

Fish have even joined the exclusive club of tool-users—something that we've long deemed (mistakenly) an exclusive hallmark of human intelligence. In 2011, a diver caught on camera an archerfish carrying a clam over to a rock and slamming the bivalve until it cracked. After eating the clam, the fish spit out the shells before continuing the hunt. Whether you want to call this "consciousness" or not, there's no doubt that it's more than mere instinct.

In perhaps the most striking finding, an Oxford University study determined that fish were able to recognize human faces. The ability to do this has long been linked with advanced brain development—specifically the presence of a neo-cortex. But fish, which lack a neo-cortex, were able to identify the one person who had fed them from a line-up of forty-four other people. They did this with 80 percent accuracy. Upon hearing the results, Australian fish biologist Culum Brown said, "the neo-cortex is not the grail of intelligence."

Nor are scientists convinced that advanced brain development is required to feel pain. Certainly the issue is disputed, with many arguing that fish lack the cognitive wherewithal to experience pain in the same general way humans do. But others note that a trout head contains fifty-eight pain receptors and that, when injected with venom, fish will rock back and forth they way mammals experiencing pain do. In another case, fish whose mouths were dosed with acid jammed their faces into gravel and rubbed them.[34]

"You should have been with us that day around the chowder kettle," wrote Walt Whitman in "Song of Myself." This quote has long evoked for me the kind of camaraderie that food can uniquely evoke. It seems downright misanthropic, in this light, to suggest that we alter the contents of the chowder kettle. But, as Whitman also wrote later in the same poem: "I lead no man to a dinner table." Our table, in other words, was our choice. And we might well ask ourselves, before we sit down to eat: What if we're not the only beings whose pleasure is at stake? With an enormous amount of evidence pointing toward the likelihood of fish sentience, it's quite possible that humans cause the suffering of trillions of creatures annually. If you ponder it, it's enough to make you eat differently.

## HEROES IN THE SEAWEED

"The most important ingredient in this soup," Larch Hanson told me, as he handed over his signature seaweed soup recipe, "is the calm mind of the cook." He looked at me with one eye squinted tightly, as if he was assessing my worthiness for this dash of Larch wisdom. Well, sure, I thought. What harm ever came from calming the mind? Who ever suffered a setback from a calming soup? Larch continued to recite the instructions for a seaweed soup seasoned with emotion: *"Relax. Pay attention. You will get exactly what you need. You do not need to worry.*

---

34. https://psmag.com/hook-line-and-thinker-caaad0afb3ff#.d6zrnae2z

*Center your breath in the heart. Trust Spirit. Put 'other' in place of 'self.'*
*Breathe deeply. Make the sound of 'ahhhh.' It is all covered."*

And it *was* all covered—but only because Larch covered it. Busting his ass, he went to sea to pull the other necessary ingredient into his boat, dry it, and bag it for me so I could, after getting it through airport security, prepare the soup at home. "I decided in my twenties to stay in the world of physical work," Larch went on. "This work keeps me healthy. You need work, just as you need love, to be happy. Freud said that."

Seaweed is (among other less obvious qualities) harvested while wet. It's virtually all water weight. Hanson effectively lifts water for a living. He dons his wetsuit, heads to his harvesting site, swims and crawls, zigs and zags his lithe frame amid large rocks, hauls the seaweed into his carrier boat, and motors the load back to shore. From there he backs a truck with a wooden flatbed to the shoreline and starts dividing his catch into dozens of aerated plastic baskets—bright orange and bushelsized—before loading the truck and taking the haul to his household compound for drying, processing, packing, and shipping.

Larch ravens across the sea after several different kinds of seaweed. A staple is alaria (*Alaria esculenta*). He describes it as "similar to wakame"—a popular seaweed used in Japanese cooking. Alaria is a product you've eaten if you've ever had miso soup in a red plastic bowl at that mediocre sushi place in a strip mall. Alaria thrives in the low surf and, says Larch, "has a very clean smell." Not fishy. The time frame to responsibly harvest alaria is brief—the narrowest for all seaweeds: the last five days in May and the first eight days in June. During this stretch, Larch labors for long hours, testing his stamina, pulling thousands of tons of seaweed from the surf daily, sleeping very little. When I asked him what he ate during this concentrated period of physical rigor, he shot me a look and said, "I'm not eating tofu." Instead, he said, he goes to a Chinese restaurant the night before and opts for fat. "I usually eat a duck."

Another popular product Larch gathers and sells is digitata (*Laminaria digitata*). Digitata requires him to ply his craft through deeper and more turbulent water. The best time to harvest digitata is evidently the day after a full moon, especially if the water is relatively calm. Nobody was able to explain exactly why this folk wisdom made sense, but several harvesters I either spoke to or read about confirmed the wisdom of following the phases of the moon. Whereas alaria requires the harvester to scramble around rocks and surf like a skittish crab, harvesting digitata, according to Larch, demands the mentality "of a rodeo rider roping calves." He elaborates, "once you manage to find a place where it's safe to work, and you get within reach of the plant, you don't want to let go."[35] Larch says the plant is similar to kombu and, once roped into the boat, has a "natural sweet smell."

Dulse (*Palmaria palmate*) is a favorite product for Larch's customers, mainly because it can be eaten right from the bag, and—for this reason—is the most commercially known kind of seaweed. It's is a crimson-colored plant that can be fried like bacon and even used in a mock BLT. It clings to rocks with what's called a "holdfast." When harvesting dulse, it's essential to cut it just above the holdfast rather than yanking it up like digitata, or peeling it from rocks like alaria. Fail to cut above the holdfast and your dulse is done. Dulse thrives in thick red blooms in intertidal zones and does best when cliffs or large rocks, as with those in northern Maine and New Brunswick, provide afternoon shade. Harvested anytime from June through September, and always at low tide (which is what sometimes sends Larch out at 2 am), dulse is probably the most versatile seaweed in terms of what the home cook can accomplish in the kitchen.

Another kind of seaweed Larch seeks is called bladderwrack. The stems of bladderwrack are studded with tiny brown cysts plumped with salt water. When it's dried, the plant has a crunchy texture. It's popular in Korean food and, as with a lot of Korean food, is often pickled. Larch began to gather bladderwrack when a faddish diet book, *Eat Right For Your Type*, made wildly exaggerated claims about its healing powers. He doesn't necessarily believe the hype, but is happy to sell healthy seaweed on the back of its popularity.

In the colder month of April, and into early May, Larch also harvests generic sea kelp. He calls it "a crisp, long, and beautiful sea elder." The

---

35. http://maineseaweedharvesters.org/kelp-harvest-season/

fact that kelp, which can grow to sixteen feet, is one of the oldest plants on earth particularly enchants Larch. He thinks that the plants have consciousness and, as such, experience a kind of collective memory. That memory, he said, should keep us humbled. How little we know, he said, compared to a species that evolved alongside the formation of the first oceans. When he hauls the kelp into his skiff, he lays them out "to let them rest," as if they had been exhausted by the transition.

The fact that there's no hard proof for plant consciousness doesn't much bother Larch. He's more at home in an imaginative world of meaningful ambiguity. The idea of an expert in anything, much less seaweed, strikes him as arrogant. "If we ever feel like we're on top of the wave," he added, "that means it's time to get off the wave." Larch the seaweed man is never swamped. But—in what is maybe his finest quality—he's also never convinced, even after four decades, that he is the master of his craft.

Seaweed is much more to Larch Hanson than a product that ensures a decent livelihood. Like the "holdfast" securing dulse to rocks, seaweed grounds Hanson's complex identity to a natural world that he values for its beauty, warmth, and health-affirming potential. "Seaweeds have admirable qualities," he writes. "They are flexible; they are tenacious; they are prolific." And at our best, so are we. This connection, he posits, is integral to the pursuit of a meaningful life, something that Larch more or less spends his time seeking.

Indeed, for Larch, seaweed, as with (his current) existence, is ultimately about connectedness—connectedness to the past, present, future, and even the afterlife. Somehow, through seaweed, "the earth's sea-blood strengthens our own sea-blood." The salt that's transferred from nature to body roots the latter to the former. "Your body is an antennae," he writes, "and your body cannot receive and comprehend the whole message from the Universe unless it contains all the trace elements of the Universe." The source of those trace elements is, of course, seaweed.

In one sense, Larch's charming spiritualism was a little frustrating. It often made it difficult for me to get empirical answers to basic questions. When I asked him how he ensures that he doesn't overharvest, he told me (without a trace of irony), "I just talk to the plants." But in another sense, Larch's brand of mysticism encouraged me to see an unexpected and bigger picture, to appreciate a work ethic that's inseparable from a life ethic, and to open myself to ideas that may not be verifiable scientifically, if only to appreciate the ways we can use myth to foster meaning in a very personal and everyday way.

For Larch, there seemed to be few boundaries between *anything*, much less labor, life, love, and leisure. For him, such divisions were distractions from some ethereal wholeness I'm fairly certain, for all my efforts, I'll never quite understand. His entire existence seemed to be one that followed a seamless, timeless, blissful flow toward wellness and comfort with the act of existing in the world.

His built environment reflected this flow. The first floor of the house was a processing facility. "When I'm not harvesting the seaweed, I'm more like a potato farmer," he said, walking around boxes of piled, bagged, dried seaweed. "I'm constantly sorting and grading my products." Upstairs was his office, where he communicated with his 5,500 clients, wrote seaweed soup recipes, and crafted moony broadsides that accompanied his goods, all delivered via U.S. Mail. And on the top floor was the kitchen, where Nina was cooking. It was here that the couple tested seaweed soup recipes (staying calm the entire time). On the other side of the kitchen was a full-sized bed.

The whole conceit of oneness with the universe can, of course, be a handful for a skeptical outsider to take in, much less take seriously. In my experience, there's always the chance that it can make a person seem like an aloof self-absorbed loon. But that's not Larch. Larch was more of an endearing eccentric who was so absorbed in his holistic vision that the question of how much of himself to reveal to me, a stranger, was moot. I could have been a potted plant and I'm not so sure Larch's behavior would have been all that different, or more generous. He never asked a single question about me, or who I was, which was fine. It kind of didn't matter.

Larch told many stories about his past. His spiritual affinity for water—an affinity that brought him to Maine—began, he told me, with his father (now deceased), who would take him pike fishing on the lakes of Minnesota. He revisits the "sacred contract" he has with his father daily and tells me that, to honor the spirit of their connection, he must activate his "heart chakra." As far as I could gather, this activation meant that, as Larch put it, "you have to surrender, and be vulnerable, and ask for help." At this moment in our interview I looked up from my notebook to find him staring out the window, in tears.

Larch's emotional spirituality is inseparable from his ecological sensibility. "An experience," he told me, "can have a seaweed feel to me." The growth in his heart was mirrored by the growth of the seaweed. His passive cultivation of the earth's underwater forest was the cultivation he undertook within the thicket of his soul. In a video he sent to me of him harvesting alaria, I noticed that his movements seemed choreographed by the waves, his body moving in elegant tandem with the shifting tides. There's no faking that kind of connection.

Given the intense nature of Larch's relationship with the natural world, he finds the concept of a seaweed farm—seaweed aquaculture is becoming a thing—to be nothing short of an aquatic crime against humanity. "The plants get old," he said. "They sit in stagnant water with no nutrients." He cringed and shook his head in mild disbelief. His inner Len Tukwilla came out when he explained that by carefully tending what long preexisted him—wild seaweed—he submitted himself, and fostered, processes mysterious and primitive, in a way that cannot be replicated on a farm. "Wild seaweed is like grass," he said. "The more you mow it the faster and stronger it grows." But, critically, the grass had to already be there. Its genetic heritage had to be Cenozoic in vintage.

Wherever the knowledge originated, knowing when, how, and to what extent to intervene in the wild underwater seaweed economy remained an essential skill to sustainable seaweed harvesting. Without restraint, one cannot ensure seaweed's longevity as a source of human and ecological health. "We've already fished out the sea urchins, scallops, and mussels," Larch said. "It could happen with seaweed." Forty years of listening to the seaweed talk, not to mention talking back, has instilled in him an intuition as sensitive as a tuning fork. It's one that's generally lost on his competitors.

Larch will rarely touch rockweed, primarily because it needs nine to twelve years to become three feet in length, at which point it can release its spores for reproduction. With alaria he waits until there are eighteen to twenty-four little vesicles between notches in the seaweed. This is a botanical indication that they've released their spores. When it comes to digitata he has learned to identify the exact shade of yellow that fringes the plant as an indication that it's time to harvest. It's all knowledge borne of close observation and long experience. Decades of harvesting have taught Larch to recognize intuitively when enough is enough. The fact that he's been coming back to the same wild harvest plots for forty years, only to find the forest beneath him become healthier and more abundant over that time, is a testament to the deftness of his touch.

Others aren't as judicious. Large commercial operations, most of them based in Nova Scotia, have come down the coast in big boats to hire underemployed local labor (Steuben's median household income is well below the national average) to strafe the seaweed beds with industrial rakes. It has rattled Larch more than a little. "They're creating chaos for me," he said, sitting on his blue yoga ball. "They're overly caught in commercial models." Larch approached his neighbors offering some of them apprenticeships in lieu of working for the big guys. He asked them, "Why are you working for these people?" Larch sighed. Then he tilted off the back of the ball, grabbing the doorframe to prevent himself from rolling into the next room.

At the center of Larch's disagreement with the big commercial guys was rockweed, the coastal seaweed that needs to reach three feet to remain viable. An Acadian based operation[36] had recently come down to Maine and started ripping the stuff out of the surf when it was only about sixteen inches high (and with indifference to the rockweed's own holdfast). A week earlier Larch left the compound to visit Maine's Department of Marine Resources and plead his case for rockweed's eco-

36. http://www.fishermensvoice.com/201610MaineResidentsVsAcadianCanada.html

logical significance. "They've got to deal with me," he said, sounding more vexed than angry.

He explained to them some critical Larch facts. Rockweed mitigates ocean acidification. It provides essential canopy for ocean life. It nourishes virtually everything under the water. It needs years to recover after a harvest. It can recover stronger—and be more available for harvesting—if the harvest is responsible. And so on. Marine Resources asked if it could see an example of the ecosystem at work. "I can't show you a full ecosystem!" he said. That would, he told me, be like showing them the working of his soul.

"How do you do that?" he asked.

This fight is active. Some wealthy property owners who want the big rakes to go back to Canada are claiming that they own the plots where the rockweed grows. Do rich people own the surf? Perhaps. If so, how much surf do they own? At what tide? There are no answers. Lawsuits are on file to address these questions in court. Larch was okay with the involvement of the fancy property owners. "Rich people need to share," he said. The Marine Resources has suggested that rockweed is a marine life no different than fish and thus fair game for the commercial harvesters.[37] "Is seaweed the same as fish?" he asked me, incredulous at such nonsense.

For now Larch abides. His access to the five-mile radius of seaweed off Gouldsboro Bay depends solely on the citizens of Steuben, who vote him the permits required to harvest. So Larch controls only what he can control. Topping that list, for all his adversity with big corporations and the state, he remains—despite their lack of interest in working being an apprentice to his mastership—on cordial terms with his neighbors.

Inadvertently, on my way in to meet Larch, I learned of this cordiality first hand. Lost, and out of cell phone range, I saw a guy working in his yard—a yard that was trashed in southern Alabama style, with six cars on cinder blocks and a toilet leaning against the house—and I asked him if he knew a man named Larch Hanson. He looked at me blankly. I said that Larch was a seaweed guy. His face then broke into a smile that said "oh *that* guy!" Yes, he knew Larch. More so, he knew

37. Rockweed: http://maineseaweedharvesters.org/who-owns-the-rockweed/

exactly where Larch danced his dance—down a dirt road, to the right, and down another dirt road, another right. "He's out there," the neighbor said, unaware that he had just nailed the perfect double entendre.

I told Larch about the neighbor. "They generally think I'm a lovely oddity," he said.

Before I left, Larch showed me a moss-covered tree in the woods behind his house. It had been damaged, probably by lightning, at some point early in the last century. It responded to the trauma by growing outwards as well as upwards, with a horizontal limb, about a foot or two off the ground, snaking through the forest like an anaconda seeking prey, getting closer and closer to the ground without actually touching it. A floating mass of hardwood vegetation. Larch looked at the tree, looked at me, and talked about the power of adversity to inspire beauty.

Then, segueing to his family tree, he brought up the topic of his grandpa. When he said the word "grandpa" it came out as "grappa." For a minute I thought I kept hearing the word for hard Italian alcohol. A tireless Norwegian farmer in Minnesota, grappa was not a drink, nor was a "grappa" a drunk. Grappa was a tireless tiller of the soil. His nose-to-the-grindstone work ethic routinely got him tossed into hayracks by unruly cattle. Grappa also talked all the time about the land around him "being lost to some corporation or another." Larch admired grappa for "vowing to be on his own," never losing his plot, never abandoning what he loved. Oh no, I thought, Larch is going to cry again. But Larch didn't cry this time. He simply paused for over a minute, looked up into the forest canopy, pointed back to the cove, and said, in his soft high voice, "I think I'll stay at this work."

## THE MORE OYSTERS IN THE OCEAN (AND ON THE TABLE) THE BETTER

"From the outside it looks so simple," said Tamar, about the fine art of farming oysters. She and Kevin were loading ice into the bed of their red pickup truck. Tamar consulted her wristwatch. With quiet urgency, she said, "hey we gotta go." Kevin double-checked the security of the skiff hitch and we hopped into the cab, Tamar sandwiched between Kevin and me. The truck lurched into gear, no chickens in the road, all passengers secure and buckled in. Weather: ideal.

When getting in the truck, I noticed that rust had chewed away the baseboards and remarked to Kevin that the salty air must be hell on local vehicles. "I use up a truck in two years," he said. "I won't spend more than $2400 on one; I figure $100 a month is about right for transportation." He hit the gas and wheels crunched over the gravel driveway. As we drove the quarter mile to the main road I had a chance to admire a large tomato garden covered in a shell of chicken wire, a pen of hens, and a thick, dense wood of maples and ferns.

There's just one landing ramp for the oyster farmers of Barnstable. It's located about four miles from Tamar and Kevin's house. As we drove to it, Tamar explained that the former owner of the land long ago granted the landing to the town under one condition: It had to serve the oystermen in perpetuity. The hard-packed low-tide beach around the loading area has subsequently become the social and economic epicenter of the town's oyster trade. It's where oyster farmers went to work, trade information, and gossip..

But, in the intervening years between the deed and the housing boom, the landscape surrounding the ramp—choice oceanfront lots— became a mushroom field of McMansions built by New England plutocrats not quite A-listed for The Vineyard. Some of these well-to-do denizens evidently didn't want grimy oystermen chugging up and down their road in their rust-eaten trucks, zooming in and out of this pristine patch of paradise, making a living off honest transactions with the sea.

"I wave at the neighbors all the time and smile and I'm as friendly as I can be," said Tamar, as we turned down the lone road toward the loading area. As if on cue, a blond woman wearing Ray Bans and a navy blue summer dress came walking up the road. Tamar waved. The woman, walking a fluffy golden retriever, stared at us like we were marauding Visigoths—or at least a bunch of roughnecks in an old truck—and did

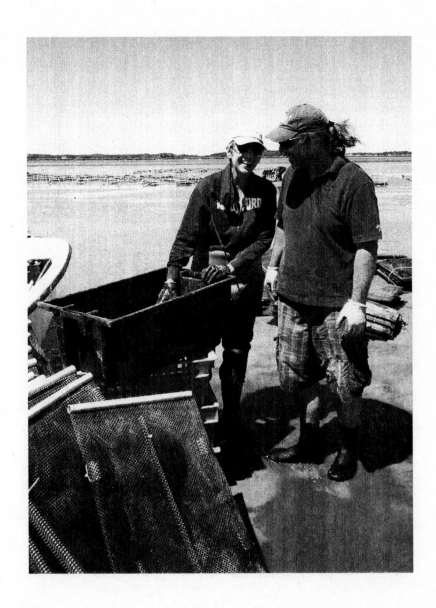

not wave back. At the landing a much friendlier vibe prevailed. Several farmers, already returned from checking their plots, were bustling about the beach in Wellingtons, shorts, and grubby t-shirts. They leaned on their trucks and boats and talked as the late afternoon sun cast a light that made everything appear emboldened, as if outlined in ink. But for us there was no time to socialize. The tides did not forgive.

I now better understood why oyster farmers gutted out their trucks every two years. As Tamar and I stood on the beach, an engine whined as Kevin hit reverse, generating the ample momentum to ram the skiff into the proper depth of water. The boat and trailer crashed into the surf and subsided in about two feet of salty sea. Tamar, now in the water, liberated the boat from the trailer and Kevin drove the truck, dripping with salt water, back onto the beach.

A puff of diesel from the outboard motor and we were off. The low tide boat ride out to the oyster acreage crossed an expanse of grey-blue water calmly coursing through thick patches of emerald eelgrass. Tamar and I sat on hard seats against the skiff's worn gunwales (actually, she gave me a little butt cushion). Kevin, at the stern, handled the outboard motor's rudder as we navigated the coastal waterway's thornier channels. I thought that, with the light and the green grass, the scenery looked like the low country of Carolina.

Water depths shifted with the tides. Kevin proceeded with a kind of nervous caution. ("From the outside it looks so simple.") To avoid the mishap—embarrassing, costly, and possibly dangerous—of ramming the boat into the ocean floor, a competent captain required a level of local aquatic literacy that Kevin, relatively new to the region, was still working to master. Fortunately, there were mentors. Generous mentors. The oyster farmers of Barnstable welcomed Kevin and Tamar when they showed up from out of nowhere. The locals were pleased to school them. Kevin and Tamar took immediate pride in being part of the Barnstable tradition. On their website they wrote, "Barnstable isn't the only place that grows great oysters, but we'll hold ours up against any other." There's solidary in the claim, a kind of loyalty to a team that seemed evident to me.

Plus, the market for oysters was so outrageously bullish that the recent arrival of another oyster farmer was hardly a threat to anyone's immediate market share. Further softening the edge of competition, Kevin and Tamar decided not to supply Boston restaurants with their oysters, removing themselves from the same market as their oyster-going neighbors. "We have New York accents," Kevin said, "so we found a Brooklyn wholesaler and decided to sell to New York restaurants alone." Finally, oyster farmers just loved being oyster farmers. Sharing the details of their craft was, especially in the current market, a genuine pleasure. Kevin benefitted in particular from the selfless guidance of one local oysterman who taught him the finer points of the trade. "We showed up from New York," said Kevin, "and the locals saw us out here and they respected us. There's some competition but not very much."

So, on the ride out, when Kevin saw a more experienced oyster farmer heading from the landing to his plot, he waved and followed. When the guy turned right from the main sea channel to go to his farm, Kevin turned left, to go to his. Now on his own, relying on several landmarks that he learned to read on the way to his farm—a white pole jutting out of the water, a pile of rocks on the shore, a red buoy—he stopped talking, deeply focused on the boat's angle to the water, trying to intuit knowledge that I sensed was not yet fully there. I held on tightly.

These markers, and Kevin's intuitions, got us to the destination. We pulled up to a sandbar the size of a football field. I tossed over the anchor and hopped out of the boat into a couple feet of delightfully cool water, wading to the sandy banks. Tamar tossed me a pair of work gloves. "There will be blood," she said. From the perspective of where we docked, this large patch of beige sand, which contained the oyster farm, looked to have been ransacked and strewn with debris. It appeared as if we'd sailed up to a junkyard studded with old bags, rebar, and pallets, if not the aftermath of a battle. But what I was seeing, and what would become much more evident as I approached the sandbar, was, alas, the operating headquarters of Barnstable Oysters.

I hate to admit this but I've been writing about food for over ten years and I really had no idea what a modern oyster farm looked like. I was envisioning something very different than what I encountered. Perhaps a bed of oysters growing from bedrock under the mud, or clinging to rocks, all them passively cultivated. And in fact it was once sort of that way—farmers cultivated native beds and, when they were ripe, chipped away at the "oyster feet" until the oysters were released. But farms have since become much more farm like since then.

As we walked closer to the beds, what initially appeared to me as a mess of far-flung debris quickly came into focus as a tightly ordered, almost sanitized, oyster factory. Stretching east to west, covering nearly the entirety of the single-acre lease, three straight lines of one hundred wooden trays (about the size of a doormat) sitting on small stilts, holding two hundred rubber bags filled with "five week old seeds"—that is, oyster seeds bought from a hatchery in Maine—stretched down the sandbar. In six hours, the whole operation would be submerged, getting fed and fertilized by the Atlantic. But for now I could have been walking in a freshly planted field of corn.

Kevin explained to me the capricious topography of the harbor's ocean floor. A hundred individual one-acre plots, plus forty-eight two-acre plots, owned by the state but leased by the town, created an agricultural checkerboard that, in terms of productivity, followed a dark logic of variable productivity that was beyond anyone's full understanding. Depending on subtle variations and undulations, depending on relative plot heights/floor depths, some plots were bathed in more nutrients than others (good), prone to different levels of algal blooms (bad), and more susceptible to forming barnacles (bad). Worse, there was little consistency as to which plots did well and which ones did not. Every year, the nutrient bath shifted. Adjacent to their current plot, Kevin and Tamar leased a second acre. "Every acre is different," Kevin said, adding that the one out of production was higher up, on a little shelf, and of lesser quality than the one he was currently farming. He was researching new oyster seeds, and packing densities, for the farm he would plant there.

Another external factor choreographing the oyster farmer's life was the tango between temperature and time. The key temp was 40 degrees. Below that and the oysters would not "bivalve," or suck in nutrients. "Over 40 and they really grow out well here," said Kevin. Harvesting happens between September and November. It's determined exclusively by shell size—some seeds take two years to reach maturity, some just one. Why? Another mystery. After November the water temperature starts dropping. It can go as low as 10 degrees. Rather than keep inert oysters in their raised beds, Kevin and Tamar transfer them to the security of a freezer. Looking out at this sprawling Levittown of oyster beds, and then looking at Tamar and Kevin (who rarely hire help), I realized that the mere thought of the task's enormity gave me a headache.

But, as with Larch, Kevin and Tamar retain a kind of comfortable affinity for productive physical labor. Plus, transferring oysters lowers the risk of disease, poaching (rare, but it happens), or the formation of sessile barnacles on the oysters. The barnacles don't harm the oyster per se, but, because they smell fishy when out of the water, they harm the oyster's marketability. The couple returns the dormant seeds back to their oceanic beds in March, just in time for the water temp to support bivalving.

The focus then turns to density. "Density is our destiny," Kevin said. Ecologically speaking he is absolutely right. As we saw with Wendy McGill's cricket can, there are big environmental points to score by producing more protein on a smaller footprint. Improving this mission is the fact that the land used, in McGill's case, is a vacant lot, and for Tamar and Kevin, the bottom of the ocean—not arable land. The issue of density is also one that Tamar frequently writes about in her newspaper columns. Every responsible food writer is concerned with sustainability, but Tamar is one of the few who—because she agrees that density is our destiny—highlights the point that one great benefit of industrial agriculture is that it has the potential (and every so often achieves it) to reach impressive densities of production.

Kevin appreciates the danger of packing too many seeds into the aerated rubber bags he loaded inside his beds: Disease can strike. It can wipe out a season of oysters in a flash. Breeding techniques have gone a long way towards making farmed oysters increasingly disease resistant, allowing for greater and greater packing densities. But still, there are limits. Oysters packed too tightly are more susceptible to the rapid spread of parasites and pathogens. Greed for density must be checked by a measure of caution. When I asked what disease most terrified them, Tamar mentioned "vibrio," a bacterium that currently gives oystermen the fantods. Kevin's current goal is 160 spats a bag—not too risky, not too safe—as the ideal balance (he was once a trader, after all). It's also a packing quotient that, in a good season, can result in 500,000 oysters emerging from one-acre plot of sand on the ocean floor. Not bad, especially if an East Coast restaurant is ransoming the creatures at three dollars a piece.

Farmers of the Wendell Berry persuasion like to talk about letting nature do the work of farming. It's a bit of a romantic notion. But oysters are in fact one of those crops for which nature does do most of the work. As we have seen, the tide comes in, the tide goes out, and the confined bivalves are nourished on the ocean's dime, with the ocean's nutrient rich soup. But for the ocean it's worth it as well. The sea benefits immensely because oysters filter nitrogen and create substantially cleaner water. Tamar said, correctly, "this is the only kind of farming that improves the environment."

Our main task was to check on the beds. Kevin and Tamar inspected them for signs of disease or stress. They looked for algae growth on the rubber bags. (Kevin noted that his new bags had diamond shaped holes rather than square ones, as his previous bags did, and that the algae accumulated much less frequently around the diamonds.) They made notes about rates of growth, eyeballing oyster sizes from different sections of the farm, noting which bags were being better fed than others.

One matter of surprisingly minimal concern—and, again, another advantage of being an oyster farmer—is that, once the oysters reach a certain size there are no natural predators. It would take a seagull about two seconds to become the proverbial crow in the corn were it not for the fact that oyster shells are a critical evolutionary step ahead of the seagull's beak: They're too hard for the seagull to drop and crack, a fact that seagulls don't need much time to discover. The other thing we were out there to do, albeit briefly, was some harvesting. Kevin looked for oysters about three inches long, maybe half as wide, and took them from various rubber bags, placing them immediately on ice. I counted around forty.

"That's a small order," I noted.

"Not for three people," he said.

Before dinner, though, came the tedium of documentation. Kevin put the oysters on ice and began to fill out little laundry tags to identify their exact source—down to the very bag. In terms of catching a food-borne illness, oysters, because they are often eaten raw, pose a higher risk than cooked foods. Regulations are thus especially layered and complex. They are multilayered—state and federal and municipal—in origin. They require mounds of paperwork. Despite their frustrating nature for many producers, the record keeping and icing requirements seemed quite reassuring to me, as was the warden who checked our small harvest when we got back to shore.

A recent white paper summarizing the state of aquaculture regulation in New England notes the excessive burden placed on oyster farmers, almost all of which are small businesses. "For small aquaculture operations, understanding the regulatory requirements can be difficult and can add significant burdens on already busy entrepreneurs." Kevin put the matter of regulatory oversight differently: "They're a *bitch*," he said. But he added that, when in doubt, "it's really not that hard to be safe; you just throw ice at it." He also said he was completely confident in their effectiveness, and ultimately knew that more was better when it came to regulation oysters. "You have to," he said. "People die."

Kevin returned to the sandbar holding a small spray pump like the one used by an insect exterminator. Soon he was roaming around the sand flats pumping jets of water into small holes in the sand. He looked like he was trying to detonate something. I asked what he was doing. Kevin said: watch, man. He pumped, and then a svelte razor clam shot from sand. He pumped. Another razor clam. He pulled them up one by one and placed them in a bowl. Soon we were all doing kind of lazy figure eights around the oyster lease, pulling razor clams from the ground, adding them to the bowl, harvesting our appetizer.

"Razor clam ceviche," said Tamar.

## MEALS

There are many reasons to explore the experiences of Larch, Kevin, and Tamar as models for the future of food. When done properly, their work has clear environmental benefits. Both seaweed and oysters enhance the ecosystem in which fish—of which we currently take trillions a year from the ocean—thrive. These products do not require unnecessary animal suffering (barring, of course, the small possibility that oysters are sentient). They are foods endowed with significant health benefits. They result from work that is remunerative and physically rewarding for the producer, work that might even lend itself to the gig-like, disjointed nature of the new economy (like insects).

Above all, their work has nothing to do with the corn-soy-land-animal complex that's at the center of what's wrong with everything food-related. All of these benefits seemed rather obvious to me, but still very much worth highlighting. It wasn't until it came time to eat these foods, though, that I appreciated something less obvious about these products, something that happened to go right to the core of my thesis about the future of food and eating promiscuously: Both seaweed and oysters court diversity. They are not center of the plate foods, but rather sides that call for other sides. They are, in this important respect, foods that push us to reimagine the nature of a meal, ask what food could be, and pursue probing questions about why we consider what we now do to be normal.

Larch sent me home with a generous bag of various seaweeds and the inspiration to make soup. "Here is a recipe for a calming soup," began his written instructions. "Relax, pay attention, you do not need to worry, your great perfection liberating you into light, is already accomplished." I actually shrugged off all temptation to be ironic and instead obeyed these words, closed my eyes and let myself "relax into the Great Presence." It felt fine. Then I went to Whole Foods. It was early October and I wanted soup for breakfast.

For thirty dollars, I left with the requisite physical ingredients. The underlying brilliance of seaweed soup is this: Seaweed is the essence of the mixture but it's an essence that can take on an endless array of accompanying vegetables. I chose barley, golden beets, carrots, burdock root,

ginger, Brussels sprouts, a daikon radish, turnips, chard, dried mushrooms, green onions, a white onion, soy sauce, miso, and, the ingredient
that is now, according to some cosmic culinary mandate, required to be
in everything: sriracha.

The soup was ridiculously easy to make. After centering my breath
in the heart, I warmed alraia, dulse, and digitata with some dried mushrooms and barley in a quart of tap water, adding soy sauce and miso
according to gut instinct. In ten minutes everything was soft and bro-
thy. Admittedly, the chopping took a while, but I did it while staying in
tune with my Trust Spirit—so the flow was pleasant. My next step was
to dump everything except the chard and green onions into the pot and
let the mess simmer for about thirty minutes. An earthy, seaside smell
emanated from the soup pot.

Once the kitchen was infused with the aroma of earth and sea, I
added chopped green onions and chard, allowing the stew to go for
another ten minutes. I finished it off with an obligatory and generous
squirt of srirachi and cut off the heat, allowing the soup to rest for an
hour. By 9 am I sat down and ate, thinking of Larch. The soup was not
only ridiculously easy to make; it was also ridiculously healthy, ridiculously tasty, and ridiculously cheap. Thirty bucks at Whole Foods sounds
like a lot of money, but keep in mind I had over ten servings of soup in
my pot. (I took about half of it to the Reeds.)

Can a pot of soup change the way we think about food? A soup
such as this one, all made possible because of Larch's harvest, steadied
the ground beneath me. During the research for my book I kept being
nagged by doubts. Did my vague vision of what the food future could
be go too far into fantasyland? Was this an exercise in utopian thought?
My hope, my strategy, was to listen closely to the people who were on
the fringes, people such as Larch, to see if I could anchor my vague utopian tendencies into something concrete. This soup was nothing if not
concrete. It reminded me that this is what eating could be: accessible,
healthy, tasty, affordable, ecologically responsible, and diverse. Thanks
to Larch and seaweed, nothing about this soup kept anyone else from
making it. And it tasted better the next day.

༼Oༀ

Tamar's table, which she was setting back at the shack, was inside a tent just outside the kitchen. Inside the kitchen Kevin was giving me a quick lesson on the best way to penetrate the outside of an oyster. I gingerly held the shucking knife, tightened my grip, found the crease, wriggled in the knife, and thrust. "There will be blood," Tamar had predicted earlier in the day. Well, as it turns out, there wasn't. I actually proved to be a natural with the oyster knife (all in the wrist), meticulous about keeping grit out of the meat, and sort of proud of my own dexterity and manual attentiveness. Still, according to the ethical vegans whose values continue to shape much of my eating (and thinking), whether I impaled my hand or not was irrelevant. Blood had already been spilled. I was eating *an animal.*

Now, a return to an important clarification: There's a temptation, at this particular juncture, to react to the ethical vegan tribe with above-it-all sarcasm. That is, to smirk off oyster sentience as a concern only a privileged lunatic animal rights nut would bother lending the mental energy of a second thought. I get the impulse, I do. But that's the easy way out. Worse, it's uncharitable. There's no point in even thinking about food reform if we aren't going to take animal suffering seriously. Absolutely none. In 2007-2008 I spent the academic year reading in the field of animal rights—not crazy advocacy stuff but hardcore and deeply thoughtful philosophical investigations. All I can say is that the experience altered how I think not only about animals and animal sentience, but also about the implications of humans eating animals that are sentient. It also ensured that there would always be, for me, serious ethical consequences for eating farmed animals.

As I've indicated, it matters if animals suffer unnecessarily for our food. It matters a lot. It's very likely that, way down the road when we know more about the nature of animal lives, we'll look back on ourselves and gasp at the depth of our cruelty. So there was no way I was going to advocate eating oysters, much less shuck them and eat them myself, if I in any way believed that these were animals that—like the farm animals we terrorize daily—understood themselves to be, as the right-based moral philosopher Tom Regan puts, "the subject of a life."

For a while I was intuitively content to rest the case, as the poet Richard Howard did in his lovely poem "Oystering," on the fact that oysters were "sealed, annealed, and brainless." But I also questioned the logic of trusting my thoughts on oyster sentience to a poet. What really tipped the scale toward eating oysters for me was an influential article published by Christopher Cox in *Slate* in 2010. Cox made a strong case against oyster sentience. But he also highlighted my long held suspicion that, for many vegans, the diet was more about an easy consistency than the reduction of animal suffering. He wrote, "If you resolve to give up foods that begin with the letter *B*, and if you stick to that for the rest of your life, you'll be mighty consistent. You'll even benefit the world by cutting out beef. But there's no good reason to avoid broccoli."

Cox then quoted Peter Singer, the Princeton bioethicist and author of *Animal Liberation*. "I've gone back and forth on this over the years," Singer said. "Perhaps there is a scintilla more doubt about whether oysters can feel pain than there is about plants, but I'd see it as extremely improbable. So while you could give them the benefit of the doubt, you could also say that unless some new evidence of a capacity for pain emerges, the doubt is so slight that there is no good reason for avoiding eating sustainably produced oysters." And this—in addition to my gut sense that an animal that lived inside a shell and never interacted with other animals could not be "the subject of a life"—was enough for me to conclude that it was ethical to eat oysters.

I shucked my last oyster and added it to the serving plate of ice. As with Larch's soup, I found myself thinking about the hidden benefit of having oysters as the highlight of a meal. Although not quite to the extent of seaweed, oysters were not really a stand-alone food. They, too, courted other ingredients to the table, thereby encouraging greater diversity in the way a steak or chicken would not do. They were expensive, for now, but that could easily change as more people oyster. They dominated nothing, but called for added ingredients.

Tamar had me chop onions and parsley for the ceviche, slice tomatoes for a salad, and deal with other small tasks. She took her own pile of tomatoes—these were all from her garden—and deftly reduced them to a pasta sauce. She prepared a cucumber salad. Kevin uncorked a couple of bottles of white wine. I recalled an old article by the writer A.J. Leibling espousing the virtue of oysters and cold white wine. Candles were placed on the table in the tent. It was a mis-en-scene appropriate for a magazine shoot.

Kevin and I sat inside the mosquito-free tent and Tamar started to bring plates of food to the table, Kevin repeatedly getting up to zip and unzip the tent to let her in and out. Teamwork. The night was cool for summertime and I could hear the pond lapping on the shore, tingling against the pebbles. The oysters were at the center of the table, surrounded by the other dishes. Everyone made a plate. Every plate was a little different.

Greedy, comfortable, I reached over for the first oyster. Kevin and Tamar watched me with anticipation. Kevin explained that the ocean nutrients "plumped up" the glistening oysters with glycogen that would mix the sea saltiness with unexpected sweetness. I wrote down the word "plumped" in my notebook, put down my pencil, and slurped. Before I even swallowed the slimy oyster, I decided that Kevin was exactly right. I looked at the oystering couple with thanks. The wind picked up. The candles flickered wildly, casting a jittery image against the tent. But they did not go out.

CHAPTER 6:

# Dead Meat

*"God created man and He created the world for him to live in
and I reckon He created the kind of world He would have wanted
to live in if He had been a man—the ground to walk on, the big
woods, the trees and the water, and the game to live in it. And
maybe He didn't put the desire to hunt and kill game in man but
I reckon He knew it was going to be there, that man was going to
teach it to himself, since he wasn't quite God himself yet."*
—WILLIAM FAULKNER, Go Down, Moses

*"I was determined to be mindful about my diet's consequences
for the world and for the many beings who inhabit it. I
aimed to confront those consequences with eyes open, to take
responsibility, to choose the path of least harm. I was committed
to finding a respectful, holistic way of eating and living, a kind of
right dietary citizenship."*
—TOVAR CERULLI, *"Hunting Like a Vegetarian"*

This is a book that, in imagining the future of food, asks readers to
chart some offbeat terrain. Still, even in the most remotely imagined culinary netherworld, the idea of a human diet altogether devoid of
meat from land-based animals seems too much to ask. Perhaps, even in
fantasyland, the notion of a meatless world is going too far. As a onetime
longtime vegan (but now, as a consumer of insects, venison, and oysters,

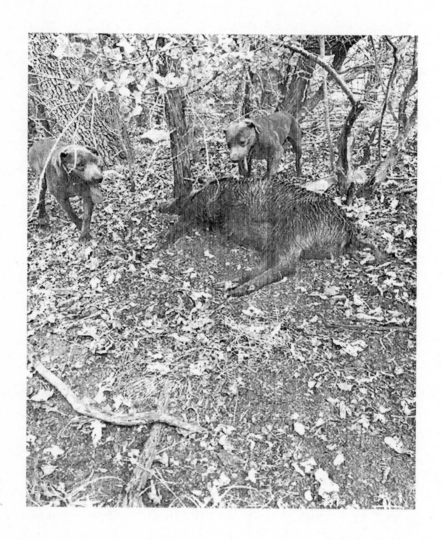

"veganish"), I closely followed the impassioned arguments made for the essential nature of eating meat. Initially, I was dismissive. *You just stop eating it; what's the big deal? Just do it and shut up.* But eventually I dove deeper into the sentiment, feeling the fuller undercurrent of our carnivoristic disposition.. However reluctantly, I eventually found it to be strong and mysterious, a force with which to reckon, if only as a cultural phenomenon not fully understood, and no longer something to ignore or downplay as selfish.

I confess that the perceived essential nature of eating meat, intellectually, continues to elude me. Humans have done a morality-driven about face on any number of activities that once seemed ingrained into our very sense of being as a species. Owning people comes to mind. So does denying women roles in the polis. But, emotionally and psychologically, there's certainly something inherent about eating animals that, even if I do not viscerally relate to it, or much understand it in my brain, makes the act central to the idea of seeming fully human. I'm not saying this is right, I'm just saying that this appears to be true for an awful lot of smart people.

It is in this more open frame of mind that, as I met the people I met to write this book, I worked to imagine a future food culture that, in some morally acceptable way, in some manner that seemed decent and thoughtful and not too much of a compromise, incorporated relatively large and obviously sentient land animals. There would, I concluded, have to be meat. "Real meat."

ᗧOᗤ

But before I get to that task, a very quick interlude. I want to weigh in—and quickly dismiss—another subject related to the meat question. There's a great deal of attention these days lavished on the ambitious idea of "lab meat." It's sometimes called "in vitro" meat or sometimes just "fake" meat. It's kind of a cool idea in concept—making meat from the cultured cells of animals—and there are many impassioned supporters of the idea. And indeed, the prospect of engineering our way around the problem of slaughter is being explored with greater and greater interest. It's undertaken by advocates who genuinely think that consumers will, for ecological and ethical reasons, accept ersatz flesh into their bodies.

But I don't think they will. In my opinion, the entire effort is a colossal gamble. Lab meat is, for better or worse, dead on arrival. The reasons for its doomed prospects aren't necessarily reasonable (but then again what about food is reasonable?). Bringing high-end technology to food production is generally a smart idea, and a great deal of our food that seems "all natural" is pretty much "all fabricated"—albeit in less obvious ways, as we have seen. So to dismiss lab meat as somehow "not real" would be inconsistent and unreasonable. For starters, it would require dismissing most of what we eat and think of as authentically the product of nature as an artifice.

In the end, though, the underlying reason for lab meat's dim prospects has more to do with something perhaps irrational but so firmly embedded in the collective human psyche that, even in the most imaginative schemes, there's no getting around it: we believe in some fundamental way that any animal flesh we eat should come from, well, an animal. Or, to be more precise, that the flesh we consume grew on the body of the animal through the process of organic growth rather in a lab through synthetic stimulation.

I'm therefore not exploring lab meat any further because I simply cannot see humans ever going so far as to accept eating meat alienated from the animal it once hung on. Perhaps someday, as with the claim that eating meat is central to human existence, I'll step back and reconsider. By for now, this is the start and finish of my take on lab meat. So: If not lab meat, then what?

## THE HUNT

Perhaps the most common alternative to eating farmed animals is eating hunted animals. About 16 million Americans hunt.[38] Ethically and environmentally, hunting is usually a better way to get meat than

---

38. http://www.motherjones.com/mojo/2013/02/hunting-demographics-charts-guns

factory-farmed animals. But is that really saying much? Is hunting an activity that could thread the needle and make its way into our imaginary future perfect food system? Confronted with the claim that hunting is a bloodthirsty and brutal ritual, which a lot of vegetarian critics think it is, the defenders of the hunt usually say something along the lines of this: If an animal lives a natural life in the wild, and is felled by a competent and ethically-minded hunter in an instant, especially if that animal is near the end of its natural life, then that animal was better off than being farmed and slaughtered. They will also say this: Hunting is a way to control invasive species. It's ecologically sound. It's a form of conservation.

I have read a great deal about hunting over the years—pro, con, noncommittal, popular, and academic. In the process, I've formed my own complicated opinions about the act of killing wild animals for food and/or conservation purposes. But these opinions were arguably compromised by one critical and nagging caveat: I had yet to actually hunt an animal myself. I didn't plan on pulling a trigger, or releasing an arrow, and taking sole responsibility for a dead sentient being. This I wasn't ready to do. But I figured I needed to at least see the act in action before determining its place in my evolving vision of what food could be. Put a little differently, witnessing every precise detail of a hunt—all the way down to the kill, the attitudes involved in the kill, and the processing of the kill—struck me as a critical prerequisite for any conclusions I might draw about the place of hunting in my idealized future food system. And so, me being in Texas, and Texas being Texas, I figured the most logical animal to chase down and kill would be a feral hog.

Smart, secretive, and reproductively insatiable, feral hogs wreak almost existential havoc among rural landowners throughout the American south, overpopulating and rooting up ecosystems with ruthless efficiency. They can, in Texas as elsewhere, be hunted year round and through any means at the ready, including firing away from helicopters, to keep them under control. They're the particular bane of cattle ranchers, who frequently offer hunters free access to their land to kill as many hogs as they can handle, and drink as much beer as they want, in an attempt, often in vain, to leave the land intact for cows to fatten on native grass, or just the native grass to be native grass.

But every now and then a wealthy landowner prefers to do the deed alone. He'll water the hounds, load up the shotgun, gas the four-wheeler ("mule"), and spend an afternoon in a lone quest for a small dose of frontier glory. So it was with Robert, a central Texas rancher I know who refused to eat meat from factory farms, rarely ate it from small local farms, and knew his way around his own property, which he managed meticulously. His attitude fell within the purview of the nature writer Christopher Camuto, who once wrote: "I've long had an odd thought that no one who hasn't killed, skinned, and butchered at least one animal on his or her own should be allowed to buy meat in a grocery store."[39]

Robert—tall, grey-bearded, in his early sixties, professorial in demeanor—preferred to eat what he killed. And mainly what he killed were deer and feral hogs, both of which overpopulated his land. I had met Robert a year ago through a friend, and I felt comfortable enough to ask if he would take me on a hunt. He agreed, but only under the condition that I grant him anonymity. Everything that follows is exactly as it happened, except for the fact that Robert's name is not Robert.

It was September and it was Texas and it was hot. As in 99 degrees hot. Robert's land extends along a pristine river in the central part of the state and the water was moving quickly enough, after a rainy summer, to bring cool water from the north. He promised a swim in the soft ribbon of blue water after the hunt. But, capturing the undercurrent of danger that would more or less characterize the entire day, he also warned me that the water moccasins had been thick of late. *I wish you hadn't said that*, I thought.

The hunt itself had to take place in the dead center of the day, under the hard blaze of a cloudless sky. For whatever reason Robert had a better success rate finding hogs between 1-4 pm, the evident witching hour

---

39. Tovar Cerulli, "Hunting Like a Vegetarian."

for the hunter. He knew enough about my animal advocacy work to realize that I was inclined to disapprove of what I might witness. So, ever solicitous, he wanted to make sure I had something to witness— because, interestingly, he thought what I'd witness would be reassuring in its literal and moral cleanliness. He thought it might possibly assuage my doubts about hunting, turn me into a weapon-wielding convert. At the least, he wanted to make my drive out there worth it.

Preparations for the outing were minimal. Fuel the mule, grab the thunderstick and ammo, pick up the hounds—two grey Blue Lacys (state dog)—at the ranch manager's house, and start criss-crossing the back roads of the ranch, in and around throngs of cedar patches and cacti, in search of a scent. Robert drove in large, looping concentric circles with minimal attempts to lessen the impact of the undulating terrain. His gun, which I held for him, was bouncing on my legs. Even through (I was told) it was emptied of rounds, the mere presence of rifle made me nervous. I didn't grow up with guns. "Most people are accidently shot by unloaded guns," Robert quipped. "But, yeah, the ammo is in the glove box. You're fine."

The dogs maintained their footing in the mule as it bounded over wild and uneven land. Their bodies rocked while their feet stayed anchored. They panted heavily, large square cur heads swiveling with bloodlust, wet black noses pitched rakishly to the sky, canine brainboxes twitching for death. Robert told me that once they caught a whiff of a hog they'd yelp like demons and leap from the bed with abandon. We'd follow. "You'll have to hold on," he said. "It'll be a rough ride."

Thirty minutes passed. Nothing. Robert, who seemed anxious that we'd come up empty, used the down time to tell me about his land— several thousand acres. Not only was it an ideal place for Robert and his family to grow up in a more natural setting, but it allowed him to indulge his interest in conservation. Over 90 percent of land in Texas is privately owned; so whatever conservation efforts take place within the Lone Star boundaries do so according to the virtuous caprice of the landowner. There are some incentives, of course. But ultimately you do it because you care about nature. In this regard, our hunt was billed an act of ecological justice.

Robert had removed invasive species and ushered in native plants and animals. He had promoted biodiversity though methods such as prescribed burns, brush management, riparian enhancement, and rotational grazing, all with the help of Dirk, his ranch manager. In a relatively brief period of time several species had recovered—namely many grasses and birds—and Robert had even discovered (and cleared flight-lines for) a bat cave. These efforts came with rewards from important conservation organizations. I wondered if he could do something about those water moccasins. Nope. Turns out they're native, too.

And then, in a hard flash, came the hit. The dogs erupted, leaping from the back of the moving mule, which was going 25 mph, and bolting like possessed underworld beasts into a dark and low-lying cedar copse. Their high-pitched yelps echoed cinematically, like screams in a horror film. Robert yanked the mule to the left in rapid pursuit, inducing something close to whiplash. We were now off road, following the yips of the hounds, who followed the scent of the hogs, who, I could soon hear, were grunting panicked snorts of fear.

One hand on the rifle, the other gripped on the metal bar above me, I was now one with the chase. For the first time, I became fully aware that I was no longer a detached observer, that this was not some silly charade without attendant risks. I was in this thing, committed, about to witness the ultimate act of violence against a non-human, but very intelligent, creature. My nerves tingled. But the visceral thrill of the hunt also clashed with my carefully cultivated conviction that animals had rights. They were, as we've seen Tom Regan put it, "subjects of a life" and, in turn, they demanded moral consideration from those able to give it. For a very brief moment, under the burden of my inner thoughts, the silence of my own doubt hammered at my conscience.

But as we careened over a pasture of chord grass I knew it was too late. This wasn't a seminar room. It was the natural world. And there were two frothing dogs baying at a terrified pig. So I did what I came to do. I did what I now told myself I *had* to do.

I went into the brush to watch Robert kill a hog.

Robert stopped the mule about fifty yards away from the commotion. The brush was too thick for the mule to penetrate without tearing us to bits. The pig's grunts had turned to piercing squeals of despair. Quickly, with the kind of focus I imagine soldiers have in battle, Robert loaded his weapon. We ran through a field of prickly pear to reach a swath of cedar that looked like a large pitched tent. With one hand on the barrel and the other on the trigger, Robert turned to me and warned, "make sure you keep a tree between you and the pig; they can be vicious; they'll charge you if I miss." *Well now you tell me*, I thought. I backed into a prickly pear that attacked my knee with a splay of thorns..

The pig, pinned by the dogs to an oak tree, wailed. The curs lunged with all the viciousness humans had bred into their bloodline. The pig's stumpy legs shuffled under a black barrel of a body spiked with greying bristles. Its head was prehistorically huge, almost cartoonish; its black eyes sharp circles of terror. Robert, who now stood about twenty yards away, raised his rifle, peered into his scope, and crouched low, staring into the brush. I prepared myself for the shot by putting my fingers against my ears. But it didn't come.

Robert held his fire. The dogs hovered over the panicked pig. He yelled at them to back off but their lust was beyond reprimand. Earlier in the day Robert had said something that surprised me: He didn't grow up hunting. He seemed like such a natural but he had never fired a gun until he bought this property a decade ago. When I asked him what kind of rifle he hunted with, he looked at me and said, "I don't really know. The one Dirk tells me to hunt with." Robert, determined to get a shot in, slightly altered his position, as if obeying some ancient law of the hunter. Again, he crouched, peered into his scope and, with the dogs on the swine like white on rice, prepared to fire. Again, I stood behind him and held my breath.

There are bubba hunters who sit in a deer blind, get drunk, and "hunt" animals lured to their coward tower by a bag of cheap corn. And then there are ethical hunters who concern themselves with the chase, put themselves at some risk, and, when the moment arrives,, make one strategically placed shot. That single shot is a point of pride. "If I do my job," Robert told me before we left, "I will need only one bullet." That bullet, if it did its job, would pierce the pig's heart and put a mercifully quick end to the terror.

Robert finally fired. His shot was a singular, cold, and echoless pop that evaporated in an instant. The pig immediately stopped squealing and tottered to the ground. The dogs backed off as if experiencing recoil. We ran to the scene. A mass of steamy blackness heaved desperate soft breaths into the brown dirt. A small patch of blood formed under the victim's left elbow. Robert had done his job. Admirably well, in fact—right into the heart went the bullet. The animal quivered, lifted its head off the ground twice, and died. I guessed that it suffered for less than a minute.

Robert went back to retrieve the mule, asking me to keep the dogs from gnawing at the dead pig. This wasn't a problem. The dogs picked up another scent and were off like banshees. I then turned around to take a closer look at the fallen beast, examining the clean but flowing wound. I walked from its backside to the front and then my heart sunk. Standing alone, with Robert and the dogs out on other errands, in this strange patch of forest, I stared with immense sadness, the kind that ached in my chest, at the animal's nippled underbelly. We'd just killed a lactating sow. The dogs were hot after the piglets.

Robert pulled up and we swung the dead sow by her legs into the bed of the mule. Before we went back to process the corpse we had to retrieve the ravenous curs, who were now yipping at a distance that sounded to be measurable in miles. For twenty minutes we searched for the dogs, who somehow went on with their wilding despite the heat and lack of water. When we finally found them they leapt into the back of the mule with the dead sow. One draped her body over the animal, as if to lay a claim to ownership. The other—her name was Tick—stood there looking at us as if she wanted something from us rather desperately. I noticed that her breathing was unusually frantic, even for a dog who had been running at breakneck speed in sheer heat for a while. Both were drenched in blood. So were we.

We reached the processing shed, and Dirk came out to inspect the kill. When he saw that it was a sow he said, laconically, in a tone that only a lifelong rancher can affect, "that's too bad." Then he and Robert exchanged a glance, implicitly acknowledging the imperative of population control, and said, in unison, "Or too good." When Dirk lowered the hatch to remove the pig, Tick, the heavy breathing dog, fell out onto his head and started writhing in a tangle of agony. His body was rubbery and apoplectic, a shaking mass of bones. He tried to stand and collapsed. Tick and the dead pig lied together on the block of cement under the shed. This poor dog was, as near as I could tell, struggling for his life.

"I think you shot him," Dirk said to Robert, without a shred of emotion.

"Maybe so," said Robert, in a similar tone of nonchalance.

Dirk turned a garden hose onto Tick and watered him as if her were a geranium. He was looking for evidence of a bullet wound. None was found. "Mighta been snake bit," Dirk speculated. At this point I had to walk away and catch my breath. I'd just watched a pig die, and I was fairly certain I couldn't witness the death of a dog without breaking down and crying. Tick clearly looked to be on the verge of death. There was blood splattered everywhere, including my shirt. And nobody around me, including Dirk's young kids, who had walked out to see what was going on, seemed to show emotions appropriate for the mayhem.

Honestly, that lab meat I just dissed sounded pretty goddamned good about right now.

## ROADKILL MORALITY
## (AND THE LOGISTICS OF ASPHALT HUNTING)

This might sounds obvious but it's an important point to note: Everything Robert and I did was carefully planned. The entire purpose of the afternoon was designed to kill a hog. The dogs were bred for the task.

The gun designed for it. The mule covered the distances that needed to be covered. The pictures I took tied a visual knot around the whole experience. Every element of the killing was, more than anything else, intentional. As a matter of morality, this intentionality cannot be ignored. It's hardly a deal breaker for the ethical nature of the hunt, but it requires a little pondering nonetheless. Driving home, contemplating the moral implications of our killing, I recognized the fact that the dead sow was the logical outcome of our carefully laid plans. I also recognized that this meant facing down a moral challenge. Namely, I had to somehow justify killing a highly sentient animal, in this case a mother, because her death provided meat and, possibly, some measure of ecological health.

Could I square these considerations without making absurd ethical compromises? We'll see. But before I make that move, I want to note how the claim to intentionality also led me to consider the opposite scenario: What if the animal was killed *unintentionally*? That is, what if we inadvertently ran over the beast and ate it? Cars and trucks accidentally reduce millions of animals every year to the degrading status of roadkill. A substantial percentage of these animals remain perfectly edible specimen after impact. Laws regarding what to do with the carcasses—mainly deer, elk, moose, and bear—vary according to state law. Some states send them to landfills, others make them into compost, and yet others feed them to zoo animals. But now, in a move that "asphalt hunters" and "freeway foragers" are celebrating, states are allowing them to be turned into dinner.

My introduction to the intricacies of roadkill morality came from a philosopher at Penn State University named Donald Bruckner. Interestingly, my introduction to the logistics of roadkill harvesting also came from Donald Bruckner. That is to say, Donald Bruckner is that kind of person: an academic philosopher who philosophizes not to make people's brain hurt but to provide a moral framework to make a little sense of his own life choices. In other words: a refreshing rarity.

First, in brief, the argument (and how Bruckner fits into it): In 2003, a guy named Steven Davis published an article in the *Journal of Agricultural and Environmental Ethics* that caused vegetarians (and vegans) worldwide to gag on their tofu. In it, he made the case that humans would harm fewer animals if they ate large herbivores rather than an exclusively plant-based diet. Davis's argument hinged on a largely unappreciated agricultural reality (one that we saw in the insect chapter): Harvesting plants kills millions of sentient animals (rodents especially)—maybe more than are killed to provide pasture-raised meat. "Perhaps," Davis wrote, "we are obligated to consume a diet containing both plants and ruminant (particularly cattle) animal products."

Davis's advocacy of beef, under the strict circumstances he posed, was compelling.. But some problems arose: His calculations were faulty; he never considered the land requirements to grow enough beef to feed the masses; and he failed to factor in the methane produced by grass-fed cattle. Still, Davis ultimately succeeded in sneaking a subversive—and ultimately productive—question into the conventional vegetarian discourse. What if there are viable ways to reduce intentional harm to animals by eating animals? The proposition surely strikes most vegetarians as absurd, if not heretically threatening to their identity. But the undeniable fact persists: Animal flesh is available for consumption without humans having to intentionally kill critters to obtain it. And that fact complicates matters for those who insist that eating animal flesh is always, ipso facto, morally unjustifiable.

This reasoning can go further. Given the extensive animal slaughter currently required to harvest plants, one might even make the case that vegetarians are *obligated* to eat unconventionally sourced forms of animal flesh in order to reduce the intentional harm done to sentient creatures. This is where Bruckner enters the picture. In an essay he published in *The Moral Complexities of Eating Meat*, he applied Davis's logic not to cattle, but to roadkill. When it comes to the factory farmed products that comprise 99 percent of the meat we eat, Bruckner writes, "We are obligated not to purchase and consume such meat because doing that supports practices that cause extensive, unnecessary harm to animals." Instead, we must eat "something else." Vegetables are an obvious something else. But so, too, he explains, is the meat lying by the side of the highway.

There's nothing hypothetical about any of this. Not only are the legal logistics of roadkill consumption in place—many states allow for the personal collection of roadkill (with some reporting requirements)—but so is a common-sense justification for doing so. Bruckner reminds us that, "Picking up road-killed animals does not harm any animals." Unlike animals churned up during plant harvests, "Road-killed animals are already dead." The upshot is that vegetarians are not only permitted to eat a little roadkill, but, according to their own "do-the-least-harm principle," they are *required* to do so. "Strict vegetarianism," Bruckner writes, "is immoral." With auto insurance agencies reporting over a million claims a year due to deer, elk, and moose collisions, eating roadkill may be a more realizable option than we think.

Bruckner took some flak over his argument. The unintended consequences of privileging roadkill as an ethically viable form of meat consumption creates disincentives to reduce the vehicular death of animals through measures such as "critter crossings." Moreover, if roadkill ever did become an alternative to factory-farmed meat—something that climate change makes entirely possible—it's easy to imagine drivers deploying their cars as weapons to run down the weak. Given that one in fifty drivers will swerve to hit a turtle in the road, according to a Clemson University study, there would be no way to know for sure, as an ethical consumer seeking roadkill, that you were eating the result of an honest accident.

But these are minor objections  at best to an otherwise powerfully persuasive argument. Bruckner—and, to a lesser extent, Davis—challenge the ethics of eating in a way that pushes us to rethink consuming domesticated or hunted flesh. For those (such as me) who argue that it's ethically unjustifiable to raise and kill sentient animals for food we don't need, but at the same time remain sympathetic to the perceived difficulties of complete carnivorous abstinence, the promise of a roadkill revolution is more than a little encouraging. It's central to the future of ethical and sustainable meat.

∽○∽

Bruckner, as indicated, breathes life into his ideas. His inspiration to harvest roadkill began with a conversation he had with a custodial worker
at his university. The custodian, whom Bruckner says he "got chummy
with," bragged about how much delicious meat he scraped off the quieter byways of central Pennsylvania. Bruckner became intrigued. "He
inspired me to go find roadkill myself," he said in a phone conversation
with me. The only other experience Buckner ever had with roadkill was
when he was eighteen and hit a deer in Ohio "A guy stopped behind me,"
he recalled, "and asked if he could take it home. I said, 'well, sure'!"

Now he decided it was his turn to collect. Bruckner clarified to me
that he has never actually hit an animal, put it in his truck, and taken it
home to eat. The road-to-table connection, he explained, was rarely that
tight. In fact he only knows one person who has done that, a friend who
accidentally hit a deer after a long day of failed deer hunting, and took
the roadkill home as a sort of consolation prize. Instead, what typically
happens is that a person will come across a dead animal hit by someone
else and, as one will, he'll freegan it. Legally, this can be done with deer
and turkeys found on Pennsylvania roadways.

How the savvy scavenger of highway flesh determines that his
bounty is safe is more art than science. It's not as if the USDA moni-
tors roadside flesh. I put this question to a doctor friend of mine (the
same one who told me I'd get hepatitis from dumpster diving) and, albeit
prone to overstatement, he had an answer: "The thing gets hit and the
shit in the thing's guts splatters all over the animal, tainting all the meat
with E. Coli that will kill you so just chill out with this promiscuous
stuff and buy your meat at the grocery store." But Bruckner the philosopher had his own ideas about roadkill safety and, I figured, the lore of
the highwayman who has not only survived, but duly thrived, on actual
roadside meat had insights that were every bit as legitimate as the mus-
ings of a medical professional with zero roadkill experience.

Bruckner pointed out that most roadkill is produced during hunting
season—October through February, when the deer are more active. The
weather is cold and the kill stays fresher longer. When breeding season
replaces hunting season, the animals roam less frequently, decreasing

their chances of roadside extermination. Relatedly, Bruckner harvests from roads frequently traveled, using a method of surveillance that further helps verify freshness. If there's no dead dear on the road on the way in to work, but there's one on the way home, you can be certain that it was recently killed and that the meat will be fresh.

Other indications are more subtle. The location of the roadkill is telling. "If it's in the middle of the road I'll definitely examine it," Bruckner said. Roadkill that the state troopers had already moved to the side of the road (in preparation for pickup by animal control) would have been out there for a longer period of time. He also noted that an injury powerful enough to kill a deer on contact would typically involve the lungs rather than the guts. "Blood coming out of the nose," he said, was a sure indication that a lung injury was the cause of death, and that the organs below the diaphragm stayed intact—so no, the meat would not be sprayed with E. coli. Further doubts about freshness or gut status could be confirmed upon evisceration. A freshly killed animal will emit a sharp blast of warmth when you cut open its chest cavity.

Ultimately it's common sense that prevails when it comes to determining what to harvest and what to avoid. "You come across deer so exploded you're like 'nope,'" said Bruckner. But he also reminded me that "the meat on a dear comes from the legs, back, shoulder, and neck and all of that is separated." He added that "if the diaphragm hasn't burst" the meat should be in good shape.

Like Robert, Bruckner did not grow up hunting. But since living in western and central Pennsylvania—deep hunting country—he has taken a sporting interest in the culture. He has attended hunts with friends and, while he never became a diehard shooter, he did pay close attention to how his more experienced friends processed what they shot. It's knowledge that, over the past six years of harvesting roadkill, he has had the chance to finely hone.

The roadkill habit started out of convenience. It was just an easier way to obtain meat. Eventually Bruckner bought a ramp for his truck in order to make the retrieval process more efficient. (Although he once tossed a deer into the back of a Subaru Forrester he was driving, doing so with the help of a highway department official who stopped to assist.) At home, he built a processing station, much like the one I saw at Arthur's and Robert's. An infrastructure of sorts emerged around his habit to sustain it.

Eventually Bruckner realized that roadkill was more than just convenient, cheap, and safe. It was also ethical. Interestingly, it was only after he started harvesting roadkill that he began writing about its ethical implications. But for all his insight into the morality of eating meat, he studiously avoided claiming any sort of moral authority on the matter. "I'm not a moral purist," he said. "My position on meat eating is not beyond moral reproach. None of us can do no harm." He knew, for example, that driving will result in the extensive death of animals. But that knowledge was not going to keep him from driving. Does that make him immoral? If so, he said, count him guilty.

Still, in relative terms, sourcing his meat from roadkill—with a single deer yielding as much as forty pounds of meat—meant not getting it from factory farms, avoiding the (possibly problematic) intentionality of the hunt, and, through the processing, better understanding the animal he chose eat. In all those qualities I saw considerable merit.

## WASHING OFF THE BLOOD

There was one specific comment that Professor Bruckner made during our interview that encouraged me to take roadkill seriously. He said: "I can't remember the last time I bought meat from a grocery store." And there it was: a revolutionary concept serving the interest of culinary promiscuity. In terms of escaping the grip of the contemporary food system, nothing could be more effective than bypassing the meat counter at conventional grocery store, spurning that tainted endpoint of an elaborate production chain that shackles us to the worst of our agricultural inheritance.

The message cannot be overstated. The sanitized meat markets of the grand American grocery chain peddle products that represent everything that's wrong with the way we eat and the system behind it. The defenders of Big Agriculture object with predictable stuffed-shirt talking points. *We've never been more efficient. We've never been more productive. We've never so effectively fed the world.* Narrowly framed, their defenses are true. But reiterating them as emblems of success obscures Big Ag's ultimate failure: Misallocating resources to produce food that harms our health and the health of the environment while treating animals who are the subject of a life as objects to be abused without consequence.

Hunting, whose rich lineage dates back to the origins of humanity, gets us around most of the problem. It evades the corn-soy-animal complex. A well-regulated hunting regimen, unless you sit in a deer blind, requires us to be assiduously active, leads to eating less meat, relies on animals who have fed themselves off nature's bounty, requires no agricultural chemicals or antibiotics, can cull invasive species in order to improve ecosystems, and connects hunters to the natural world. All good. There is, as a result of these differences, no question that hunting is a much better way to acquire meat than to buy meat grown on a "farm," or even a real, old-fashioned local farm.

But then there is the brutality—an intentional brutality—that popular dialogues on food and farming either ignore or too easily rationalize with excuses rather than justify with real arguments (excuse #1: animals hunt animals so it's moral for us to hunt animals). Most people who hunt (at least in wealthier parts of the world) do not have to hunt. Robert and I did not, for any good reason, have to be out there chasing a feral pig (aside from me needing material for my book). I understand that justifications for doing so might be virtuous. To wit, one of the best essays in favor of ethical hunting, from a writer named Tovar Cerulli (he calls himself a "mindful carnivore"), explains it so well I want to quote it at length:

*I wanted to feel more a part of the land, to see differently, to sharpen my attention, to feel more like a participant in nature and less like a spectator. I wanted to engage with and better understand the local ecosystem, the wooded ridges and valleys that the white-tailed deer and I both call home. I sensed that hunting might help me establish a different relationship with the land, a sense of belonging, a kind of communion. Communion through hunting? A few short years earlier, the notion would have stirred suspicion in my mind and heart......* Now, *though, I knew hunters – both men and women – whose respect for nature was no mask. Their compassion for animals and their concern for the health of the planet were undeniable. They took to woods and fields, as hunter-feminist Mary Zeiss Stange has put it, "for the same inner reasons they always have: for food, of course, but also for connection, and for knowledge about what it means to be human in our complex and increasingly fragile world.*

I like it. I get it. It's a generous and virtuous assessment of a morally complex way to obtain meat. Yet, there were those piglets—those piglets whose mother Robert, with me as co-conspirator, shot through the heart. I thought about them for days after the hunt. On one of those days, while driving into work, I actually cried. You can roll your eyes at my sentimentality, but I did. I think pigs are nasty animals. But still, no matter how many "MMMM Bacon" shirts we print, I know that they feel their lives. So there's that reality to face. There's that reality to work into the other side of the invasive-animal equation: the intentional suffering we caused. Back when Tamar and Kevin took me oystering, Tamar joked "there will be blood." But this time there really was blood. A lot of it. And it was, literally and figuratively, on my hands (and my arms, my clothes, my neck). And it was there because of an intentional choice I had made.

But roadkill was different. Roadkill, which is basically *unintentional hunting with a vehicle*, is hard to dismantle on any front. It clears the same hurdles that hunting does, at least when it comes to avoiding the evils of meat's agribusiness racket. Likewise, unless the driver is a psychopath who goes out to purposefully run over animals for dinner, the method of acquiring the meal, while certainly brutal for the animal involved, does not aim to do anything else but get you from point A to point B. It's hardly unreasonable to imagine a state agency or private corporation created to collect, clean, and process roadkill before testing it for safety and selling it to consumers. We'd eat a lot less meat. But we'd also eat more kinds of meat, none of it would be farmed or intentionally harmed, and, with proper oversight, it could be safer than the factory fare that comprises most of what we currently consume with so many terrible consequences.

♡○○

Robert was still learning to process a pig. But in order to ensure that I saw it done expertly, he asked Dirk to demonstrate. Dirk, in all his terseness, grabbed a hand-sized whetstone and started sharpening his tiny pocketknife. *He was going to butcher a 200-pound pig with a pocketknife?* Robert nodded at me as if to say, *amazing, right?* Truth be told, it kind of was amazing. With Tick, the possibly dying dog, finally starting to recover a little, but still unable to stand up, Dirk cut into the dead pig's backside, just behind its head, and executed a firm downward slice. The sound was scratchy, like he was tearing burlap.

The incision, extensive as it was, did not produce more blood. Instead, it exposed a waxy layer of hard white fat. Dirk, who now worked with all the delicacy of a surgeon, cut under the skin about six inches away from the spine, separating skin from fat, and folding the flaps of hide over the animal's flank. Rather than disgust, I found myself contemplating the indignity of the dead animal's posture. An hour earlier she was digging up grubs in a cedar copse. Maybe she was happy. Maybe not. But she had emotions. Now she was a dead body, face down on a patch of cement, arms and legs splayed at right angles to her body, looking like she had been unzipped from the back of the neck to the tail, which. In a way, I guess she had.

All this effort for a single pig. This thought led me to explore the conservationist claim that supposedly justified the hunt. When I pushed Robert to explain how shooting one pig served the agenda of population control, he equivocated a little. I recounted some research I'd read arguing that hunting feral hogs can actually worsen the problem. Because the animals are so smart, they reliably associate the region where a shooting took place with danger and, wisely, find new places to live. Many conservationists think that shooting hogs thus leads to more hogs moving to more places. They now populate the entire lower forty-eight, in large part because hunters do what a leaf blower effectively does to leaves—scatters them, making them someone else's problem.

Robert eventually conceded that isolated hunting was probably sending more hogs to his neighbor's ranch. He also conceded that, to really make a dent in the hog population, he would have to bring in heli-copters, tracking devices, and semi-automatic thundersticks. Another hunter I knew agreed with this assessment. The lone hunt could be counterproductive. He told me that he knew hunters who were experi-menting with rifle silencers, testing the proposition that it was the noise, more than any other factor, that forced the hogs to migrate elsewhere.

After removing a few pounds of meat off the back—"the backstrip" they called it—and stuffing it in a Ziplock bag, Dirk, who was pressed for time (it was his daughter's birthday and they had a party to prepare for), convinced Robert that the nominal amount of additional meat they'd get from gutting the carcass wasn't worth the mess. "Skip the loins," sug-gested Dirk. I can't say that I was particularly upset about not getting to see a dead pig's guts spill to the concrete floor. Robert also took the decision in stride, eager to drive the carcass out to a field near the river where native turkey vultures—who Robert, a bird enthusiast, had a spe-cial interest in—would consume the animal. As we drove away, I saw Tick, wobbling around, unsteady and confused, like he was drunk. But he was up, and alive. The consensus was that he had, during the chase, badly overheated.

We dumped the dead animal in the pasture without ceremony before heading down the hill to the river for our swim. The water was clear and the day's heat was dissipating under a light breeze. After checking the riverbank several times for snakes, I sat on a rock and started to change into my suit. Just as I was cinching up my trunks, a wild sprawl of naked white flesh, legs kicking into the air like Tarzan, a body thrilled with the sensation of motion, careened overhead. I looked up to see Robert, rid-ing a rope swing in all his glory, on his way into the cold river. He rose up on the swing, hovered for a moment, smiled, and let go. When he hit the water a kettle of vultures exploded into the amber sky, casting a brief shadow over our freedom. And then they flew away.

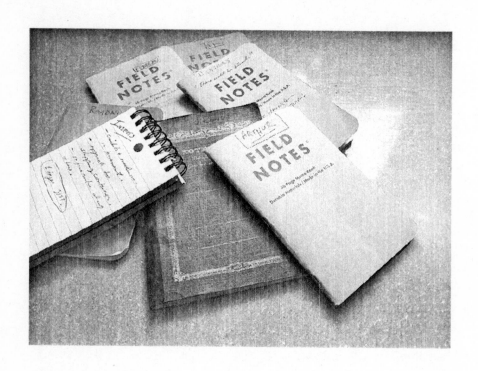

# Becoming Promiscuous

## A TOUR THROUGH THE TYPICAL AMERICAN GROCERY STORE

On the day before Thanksgiving, 2016, I entered a grocery store in East Texas, about seventy miles outside of Houston, to pick up a few last minute items for the holiday gathering at my in-laws' ranch house (Saran Wrap, edamame, drinking water, avocados). I left the store—a standard place—not only with the requisite goods, but also with a vivid reminder of why I wrote this book.

After walking in and immediately encountering a multi-tiered rack of frosted donuts, bear claws, another rack of candy bars (and, later, not a single ripe avocado), I called the house and said I was going to be a while. I decided to take myself on a tour the periphery of the grocery store—the very place where food experts tell us to stick to when we shop for food—and record every option that was available on the eve of America's most important annual culinary event. This impromptu research project proved to be a telling experience, one that began with curiosity, progressed to dismay, and culminated in outrage. This store, this all too typical store, came into focus as a relentless manifestation of our victimizing trap. It's exactly where we had to locate our food problem and, somehow, in some way, fix it.

After passing the checkout line, I encountered a large table holding pecan pies, bundt cakes, apples pies, and "Christmas Tree cakes." Behind the table was a stand of boxed Coca-Cola cans stacked like Lego pieces in a freezer. This was next to a big basket holding boxes of Stove Top stuffing and cake mixes. To the right, along the south wall, was a produce section that stretched maybe forty feet in length. The basic items you'd hope to be there were all there: carrots, broccoli, Brussels sprouts, avocados (all rock hard), spinach, lettuces, and fresh fruit (apples, bananas, oranges, and so on). They were tired looking but, at least, available.

In the middle of the aisle was some more good stuff— bins of nuts, potatoes, onions, and yams—but situated alongside these offerings were bins of (more) Coca-Cola, Sprite, and enriched dinner rolls. On the shelf across the aisle there were about thirty feet of processed bread (98 percent of it in the Wonderbread vein, the rest whole grain), hot dog and hamburger buns, Apple bear claws, oatmeal cream pies, Snowball cakes, more frosted donuts, Twinkies, honey buns, fudge rounds, and—within a few feet of the real bananas—banana marshmallow pies. Finally, just in case you missed it earlier, more Sprite.

From there I moved to the back wall of the store, which began with the obligatory thirty-foot case of lunchmeats. This display included processed bologna, turkey breast, ham, roast beef, and salami followed by combination "loafs" going by such names as "liver cheese" and "ham and cheese loaf," which had dots of yellow amid the puffy pink meat. One thin slice of these loafs, I observed, contained about 30 percent of the recommended cholesterol for the day, in addition to 20 percent sodium and 15 percent fat. Then came the "lunchables"—marketed as pre-packaged school lunches. Regarding these lunch options, one could choose from main meals such as nachos and cheese, hot dogs, pepperoni pizza, or mini-burgers. To round out the meal, they came with small Kit Kat bars and a boxed fruit juice. Adult options at the end of the cooled display case included huge chicken drumsticks, shredded pork, meatloaf, bacon and cheese mash potatoes (in a small bin that, if you ate the entire thing, would provide 100 percent of the recommended fat intake for the day). Interrupting my journey down this path of processed meat was a bin containing massive bags of corn chips.

I decided to negotiate the back row of the store in a zig-zag pattern. On the aisle opposite the processed meats one could buy tortillas, sausage seasoning, boneless chicken "wyngz," grilled chicken wings, popcorn chicken (all of this chicken is frozen in plastic bags), honey-BBQ glazed wings, and crispy chicken strips. At the bottom of the freezer, on a small shelf, you could bend down and hoist up six-pound cans of hominy (two for five dollars). Next to this was a display of canned cream of mushroom soup, beef stock, bags of sugar, jars of corn syrup, evaporated milk, chocolate chips, pumpkin cake mix, vanilla wafers, salt water taffy. Back across the aisle, I noted pork "cracklins," pork butt roast, stew meat, beef ribs, boneless chuck, brats, pork chops, catfish fillets, and five-pound tubes of ground beef. On the other side there were cases of Bud Light, beef jerky, summer sausage, salami, canned green beans, cornbread mix, potato chips, canned tomatoes, saltines, "two-alarm chili kit," salsa, Velveeta, corn chips, yet more Coca-Cola, chocolate covered raisins, Sprite, microwave popcorn, Fanta, twenty-four-ounce bags of cheese puffs, Dr. Pepper, Pepsi, sugar cookie mix, and potato chips.

Dairy products dominated the rest of the back of the store. The section without cheese included milk of every fat percentage, almond and soy milk, creamers, chocolate milk, sour cream, French onion dip (with bacon if you preferred), yogurt, eggs, whipping cream, guacamole, salsa, shredded hash browns, egg whites. Then came ten feet of fruit juice—mainly orange, grape, tropical punch, and apple. After five feet of butter and butter like products, including squeeze Parkay, came cookie dough, butter rolls in tubes, cinnamon buns in tubes, pizza crust in tubes, and biscuits in tubes. The last section of the back of the store was a case with processed cheese of every imaginable formation: whipped, hard, soft, shredded, and creamed.

Rounding the corner to the side of the store on the opposite end of the produce section revealed a corresponding wall of oatmeal (dried and instant), granola bars, vanilla wafers, fruit roll ups, pop tarts, bags of candy, and a massive display of cereal, all of it sweetened (with the exception of the shredded wheat). On the other side of the aisle: sports drinks and more juice—Gatorade, Powerade, Kool Aid powder, juice boxes, gallons of tropical and grape juice, V8.

My return to the front of the store brought me back to where I entered, but not before sending me bobbing and weaving amid table after table of miscellany, plus a little restaurant. The little restaurant served hash browns and fried chicken. Otherwise there were corn chips, puddings, pop tarts, gummy bears potato chips, cupcakes, dinner rolls, Danish bear claws, jumbo honey buns, hard candy (including candy canes), chocolate covered cherries, more candy canes ("believe in Jesus" brand), caramel popcorn, blocks of cheese, smoky bacon cheese balls, Coca-Cola, cookies, pork ribs, gallons of Hawaiian punch, summer sausage, sausage casings, and, last but not least, bullets.

And this was just the periphery of the store.

We are the products of our environment. This grocery store is our environment. It's a venue so commonplace, so entrenched in our dietary landscape that we rarely think to question its legitimacy as an institution. It feeds us and, as a result, we're happy to patronize it. It promises to nourish and please us and so we trust it. But as I toured this store's circumference, a different kind of reality set in. The feelings that welled up as I slowed down to record items I typically walked passed without taking a second look went from inquisitive to despairing to angry. What have we done to ourselves? Why have we accepted this institution as normal (or even as a measure of success)? I thought back to the Reeds—*of course they became overweight*—and how hard they are working to avoid the traps within this insidious and degrading kingdom of food.

Obviously, given this endless litany of junk food (with a few exceptions), it's no surprise that we are chronically overweight and suffering from chronic lifestyle diseases. Nor is it any wonder—given how much of what I catalogued was rooted in the corn-soy-sugar-animal complex—that our environment continues to bear the burden of this energy- and water-intensive misallocation of agricultural resources. The number of animals that suffered to make these foods available was, we should also note, beyond measure. And yet, lured by the pleasure of a pop-tart and a Coke, very few people ever wonder if this well-lit place, this generic grocery store stocked with comforting abundance, might be the source of tremendous human and animal suffering.

My main goals in light of this experience have been at least three-fold. I wanted to: a) Imagine an ideal future food system, one that has little to do with how we currently produce and consume food and one that is optimally diversified to the benefit our bodies, our environment, and the welfare of animals we currently domesticate for food; b) Spend time with outliers who were already pursuing these ideals through agricultural principles and methods of production that pushed us in brand new directions, observing how these renegades were laying the foundation for a future food system that allows us to eat a diversity of nutrient dense, low-impact foods with admirable promiscuity; and c) Present my findings in a way that makes them seem both peripheral to what we know about food reform but also inspiring, broadly radical but not narrowly ideological. In essence, I wanted to highlight eccentric approaches to food that, for all their weirdness, were achievable for us all, but by no means achievable in a way that has been systematically attempted.

This is not a policy book. People who want clean policy answers to the problems I've addressed have already asked me: How do we do this or that? And my answer is *I'm not sure*. I pursued my pie-in-the-sky vision without any claim to knowing how to fulfill it (but also confident that there are people out there able to engineer solutions) but assured that whatever "it" was needed to be articulated and addressed with creative imagination. This book is, therefore, essentially a case of me channeling a decade of thinking and writing about food into a realistic fantasy of what food could be rather than a case of harping too much on what it now is and how we can make immediate changes to solve immediate problems.

That said, I want to end by bringing the reader to the brink of turning ideals into action. I will do so by first presenting a vision of what the future grocery store—the crucible of our culinary promiscuity—could look like. I basically want to envision the opposite of today's grocery store and, in turn, propose what consumers can do to nudge our food system in that better direction, one that makes such a reformed shopping experience conceivably possible. We have, through the men and women I have profiled, seen examples of what the periphery of the food system is like. We have seen glimpses of the future. Now we can start thinking about how to bring those peripheral cases to the center and establish private eating habits that might have public consequences for the most fundamental of humans acts.

## PRINCIPLES

Before touring the grocery store of my imagination, we should revisit the principles uncovered by my adventures. As should be clear, I ended up feeling tremendous respect and admiration for the subjects I interviewed and shadowed as they went about their work. From each person I absorbed distinct principles that were directly relevant to a responsible future of food, principles that, if widely embraced, would, I am sure, enable us to escape the pitfalls of the past and think in genuinely reconstructive and optimistic terms about the human diet.

After documenting (via the Reeds) what's required to escape the trap of obesity and the food system behind it, I began with Arthur Haines, whose intimate knowledge of nature's uncultivated culinary potential highlights the hidden diversity of plants (mostly) and animals that exist beyond the bounds of conventional agricultural production. I juxtaposed his story with that of Cibus's Greg Gocal and Dave Songstad, plant geneticists whose gene editing technology offers the potential to improve upon—and widely expand—the natural diversity that Haines exploits to include any food for which we have a seed stored. Cibus has the means to make plants more nutritious, less resource intensive, and capable of growing under a wide range of climatic conditions. The marriage of these ambitions—Haines emphasis on diversity and Cibus's precision to achieve traits supportive of promiscuous eating—seems essential to pioneering a varied and nutrient dense diet of plants and animals.

From there I explored Wendy Lu McGill's insect farm—as well as her struggles in getting her operation up and running. Insects are the most abundant, diverse, and healthiest animals on the planet. We could be eating thousands of types of insects and we would be much healthier as a result. Insects are cheap to raise, have minimal ecological impact (especially next to traditional animal agriculture), and represent a large spectrum of tastes and textures. McGill's start up, forged in a re-used shipping container, suggests how the future food system could also become more accessible to both producers and consumers. With insect feed coming from other forms of food waste, mainly spent brewers' grain, and insects able to convert all of that feed into edible flesh, we are looking at a nascent industry with a prominent role to play in replacing our reliance on protein from land based animals that are sentient and require tremendous amounts of processed feed to reach slaughter weight. Insects are, moreover, an every person's food, the ideal grub of the street. If you think that the idea of eating them is gross, just look at the ingredients in most of the food I recorded at my East Texas grocery store. Is it that crazy to think that most of us would take a well-prepared and crunchy insect burger over a slab of liver/cheese loaf?

Dumpster divers further reiterate this critical emphasis on widespread access to food while espousing a dietary philosophy that, by virtue of being rooted in consuming waste, is refreshingly open to experimentation. The freegans I met—especially Karen and Dave—dug through trash for food. While that sounds desperate and stunt-like, it was in fact neither. The dumpster dive, particularly in places such as New York City, yields more calories than the average team of divers can consume on the spot. Accordingly, freegans find and share food; they think about food in communal terms. It's integral to their work. They host dinners in public and private spaces. They bring excess food to community centers and whenever possible offer food to the homeless. The underlying mission might be to opt out of capitalism, but the takeaway is more usable realistic: You can merge your dietary habits with ideals. And if those ideals happen to center on eating promiscuously and democratically, freeganism hits the mark. Freeganism, finally, was less "down with the man" and more about denying food's power to mark class distinction. No other group of people I spent time with made me think more about the social consequences of eating in conventional restaurants, which are, when you think about them, one of the most conspicuous and exclusive forms of achieving distinction (or not) available to us, not to mention centers of waste production that freegans rightly abhor. After my evening digging through trash with freegans, I effectively stopped eating at fancy restaurants and, on the rare occasion when I did eat out, I sought out food trucks serving honest food under eight dollars an entrée.

Consistent with the move away from raising land animals for food is a turn to the bounty of the world's oceans. Given the fact that the vast majority of the earth—70 percent—is water, it makes sense for humans to reduce our reliance on land and turn more to water for our food. To the extent that we have done so, however, the outcome has been an ecological and ethical disaster. The global fishing industry has, through brute force technologies, depleted the oceans of fish stocks. Three people I interviewed—Larch, Tamar, and Kevin—approach the ocean in an entirely more responsible manner. By sustainably harvesting seaweed and oysters, they accomplish more than the current agricultural goal of doing the least harm to the environment when it comes to producing food. They improve the environment. They do so, moreover, without harming sentient animals, thereby enhancing their own connection to the landscape, while providing incredibly healthy food that inspires greater creativity with more ingredients in the kitchen.

In the past I've worked under the assumption that there could be no land-based animals eaten in a just food system. This was an easy assumption to uphold when I surrounded myself with vegans. But the more I talked to thoughtful meat eaters, the more unrealistic this stipulation seemed. These conversations led me to explore the possibility of including meat from land-based animals in my imagined future food system. Hunting was a logical starting point. As for my conclusion on that option (at least based on my own experience hunting a feral hog), the answer is: it's complicated. But I think there's a good argument to be made for eating hunted invasive species, of which there are thousands. Easier to justify is roadkill. It sounds a tad insane, but if the college professor I interviewed can source his meat from the highway, there's no reason that the rest of us couldn't entertain the idea as well. Bottom line:

the future of food will include meat, and a decent amount of it. It will just have to be very different from the narrowed range of meat we eat today. Without exception, it should not be domesticated for the purpose.

To recap, the principles embraced by my subjects can be boiled down to about a dozen characteristics. The food of the future will have to be radically diverse, easy to produce, low impact on the environment, accessible to all, respectful of animal sentience and welfare (at least in terms of intentional harm), transcendent of the categories through which we now currently think about food (organic vs. conventional, natural vs. GMO, local vs. global, and so on), ecologically ameliorative (when possible), oceanic (but no fish), nutrient dense, high tech, home kitchen rather restaurant based, and rooted in systems of production dedicated primarily to producing food for people to eat directly—a strange thing to stipulate, but, alas, necessary).

## THE GROCERY STORE OF THE FUTURE
## (OR, EAT MORE THAN KALE)

The principles articulated above are the opposite of those informing the East Texas grocery store I scrutinized on the eve of turkey day. How, we might ask, would these principles be manifest in the layout of a grocery store? What would that kind of shopping experience look like? The starting point for exploring this fantasyland of food has to be a fundamental shift in agricultural resources followed by two caveats. The fundamental shift in resources would require taking the 210 million acres of land that are currently used in the United States to grow corn, soy, and hay and swap it out with the fruits, vegetables, nuts, and legumes grown on fifteen million aces of land. The two caveats are that a) the fifteen million acres of corn and soy would be phased out for a transition to foods grown for people to eat as soon as possible; and b) the 210 million acres of diverse plants would seek increasingly less traditional agrarian modes of production—with indoor and greenhouse being options—and the inclusion of cutting edge biotechnology. In other words, the less the system looked like traditional farming, the better.

This transition would be mirrored in the offerings of an everyday grocery store. The entire center of the store—given that 210 million acres—could now be an open market of fruits and vegetables numbering in the several hundreds rather than, as today, in the dozens. These plants could be engineered to be nutrient dense and ecologically low-impact. The store would carry the conventional fruits and vegetables that we're already accustomed to seeing in grocery produce section (but now there would be dozens of varieties of each). But, in order to reduce waste, the store would also favor plants that do not rot quickly, such as root vegetables, Brussels sprouts, squash, cauliflower, fiddleheads, sweet potatoes, onions, yams, cassava, lotus root, beans, chickpeas, nuts, lentils, dried berries, rice, quinoa, kamut, freekah, bulgur, spelt, millet, amaranth, teff, barley, and farro. To avoid a tedious list highlighting the vast diversity of these foods, I'll only note that there are about thirty edible grains grown today, thirty-two varieties of potatoes from Ireland alone, hundreds of bean varieties, dozens of lentil types, thousands of types of rice, dozens of commercially available edible roots, and hundreds of edible nut and seed species. These crops—all of which could be grown abundantly and with relatively low inputs in the United States or Mexico (and most of which could be sold in bulk)—would form the foundation of the grocery store of the future. We would do most of our shopping in this expansive arena.

A special section of the plant-based center of the store would focus on green vegetables, particularly leafy greens. These crops are more perishable and should therefore be purchased from wholesalers with greater frequency and in lower quantities in order to avoid waste. Many of these crops—broccoli, cabbages, lettuces, arugula, mustard greens, collard greens, bok choy, kohlrabi, watercress, chicory, chickweed, Chinese cabbage, samphire, rare chard varieties, spinach, herbs and, of course, kale—could be grown hydroponically, year round, and indoors, all on a small-scale. Again, this, too, could be done as a part time endeavor in the gig economy.

At Texas State University, Nicole Wagner and a team of researchers are paving the way for this kind of piecemeal production. They recently designed an experimental agricultural pod combining hydroponics with a shipping container (you get the sense that these containers are going to play a huge role in food's future). The idea is brilliant, elegant and wildly adaptable: Create a system whereby a finite amount of nutrient rich, constantly recycled/filtered water fed plants inside the can, with all energy needs—namely temperature and artificial light—controlled (as we saw with McGill's insect farm) by solar panels. No soil required. Wagner and her team are working with a million dollar grant from the USDA to make this system foolproof and replicable. Along with the grains, tubers, beans, roots, and nuts, hundreds of types of green vegetables grown in this fashion could create a consumer landscape that encouraged food shoppers to graze the open market much as Arthur Haines grazed his open fields.

The next section of the store would focus on dried and pickled foods sold in bulk and used mainly as the basis of soups, sauces, and stews: namely seaweeds, algae, and mushrooms. All eight of the major seaweeds now used as edible food by humans would be available in dried form. They would be immediately usable upon hydration to make soups, fill sandwiches, and adorn salads. Of the thousands of known edible mushroom varieties, the grocery store of the future should be expected to carry—both fresh and dried—hundreds of them. As for algae, farmers currently cultivate it for use in biofuel. But future uses will likely center on supplementing nutrient rich cooking oils, a promising development for both human health (as omega 3s and 6s are well balanced in algal oil) and the environment, as algae farms (the most important one in the U.S. being Harlingen, Texas) sequester carbon dioxide, thereby mitigating greenhouse gas emissions. One tasty non-oil type of algae we could eat regularly are sea grapes, which look like tiny green lentils strung together and are extremely high in vitamins B, A, C. In any case, these foods are healthy, non-perishable when dried, and extremely versatile in the kitchen. It's the kind of versatility, moreover, that encourages the use of many ingredients, thereby promoting the objective of eating promiscuously.

Moving into the meat section, a large part of the grocery store of the future could be dedicated to an abundance of insect species. As we have seen, there are over 2,100 varieties of edible insects. They can be prepared in a number of ways, but one might envision buying them in bulk and snacking on them the way we snack on nuts, including them in smoothies, frying them to use as garnish on salads, and making burgers or tacos out of them. They can also be purchased in flour form, from which we can replace wheat flour with cricket flour, as many bakeries are starting to do. Cricket pancakes with maple syrup? Cricket biscuits? An emphasis on insects would also allow consumers to support more local farmers than is possible with conventional animal agriculture, as land requirements are minimal and opportunities to explore niches within the world of insect production are abundant (with 2000 or so options). Instead of building so many storage facilities (which seem to go up everywhere in Austin), how about renting that space to insect producers working out of small, indoor venues? Growing insects could become an indirect way to support local breweries as well, as they could now sell their waste to insect producers to use as feed.

Replacing the more conventional meat counter would be a much different and more varied kind of counter, one stocked with government-inspected roadkill; hunted and scavenged invasive species; and shellfish such as oysters, mussels, and clams. These offerings would provide less meat than we are now accustomed to having. But that's fine because, by all accounts, we should be eating less meat (eating less meat, in turn, would foster a broader range of plants). We should also be eating more types of meat. The range of possible options is, when domesticated animals are eliminated, much broader and more exciting than the chicken-beef-pork-salmon complex to which we now limit ourselves. Imagine choosing among feral hog, jellyfish, venison, raccoon or possum sausage, zebra mussels, pike, Burmese python, freshwater clams, sea snails, rock pigeons, European starling, veined rapa whelk, swamp deer, and brown tree snakes. Perhaps one day we might open our minds and palates up to nutria, rats, and shelter dogs about to be euthanized. To the extent that we can preserve these meats by smoking or jerking them, all the better. This need for preservation is especially important for oysters, which we should be producing in higher quantities but have a split-second shelf life and, as a result, should be, more often than not, smoked and cured in oil rather than served fresh.

Finally, the ring of the grocery store would provide minimally processed specialty items such as cooking oils, chocolates, tofu, alcohol, breads, hummus, spices, salts, eggs, and coffees. Especially significant for this section would be the ongoing proliferation of micro-brewed beer, a decentralized industry that would provide the basis for insect feed. (In the last twenty years, microbreweries have grown from about 200 to 4000). As for the eggs, these would only be pasture-raised and rare, available from farmers who harvested eggs from hens who were kept by farmers as a supplemental aspect of their operation, primarily to restore grasslands rather than produce meat. Plus, chickens would require a very small amount of soy-based chicken feed, which could also be used by insect farmers who feel that their stock needs more protein. As Wendy McGill observed of her stock on the rare occasion she uses chicken feed: "they get fat really fast."

This proposed arrangement might seem so different from what we're used to that the prospect of achieving it seems totally unreasonable. But at least two considerations should prompt us to resist such a conclusion. The first is that the expanded range of ingredients offered at this sort of market would make it very difficult to eat badly—as in unhealthy. Just as I had to hunt for a handful of healthy ingredients at the East Texas grocery store I visited, one would have to do the same for the unhealthy ones at this imagined grocery store. We would, in other words, largely be able to walk into a grocery store, buy food, cook it and eat it, and—as a direct result of the food itself—have a healthy diet. No longer would people such as the Reeds have to fight their way out of the trap set by our food system—a system that, ironically, is always touting its access to choice. Second, by virtue of the diversity built into the system, all the other goals that leading reform efforts seek to accomplish—for food of the future to be sustainable, accessible, abundant, and humane—would follow this transition toward diversifying our food system by eliminating the corn-soy-sugar-animal complex.

As indicated, I've no concrete plan for how to do this. There's no policy map for enacting whatever structural changes would support promiscuous eating. But I do know that, on some level, change starts with individuals supporting that change in both theory and action. Regular consumers might think that there's little they can do to reform something as massive and powerful as the food system, especially along the radical lines that I suggest. That is, it's easy to think that our lives are too distant from the people I've profiled, and that the people I have profiled are simply too niche-oriented, to engage in meaningful change. But this is not so. What follows is a list of ways that we can all start bringing peripheral ideas about eating promiscuously to the center of our lives, introducing and fostering ideals and habits that are essential to reform, better health, and greater sustainability. They are behaviors that, in the course of researching and writing this book, I have personally embraced as emblematic of "the bonobo diet."

—Make eating different foods—even foods you have never heard of—a daily priority. At one vegan macrobiotic place in Austin where I routinely eat, I will often consume, in one meal (for nine dollars), over thirty different types of plants. Many of these meals have included plants that I once never thought to eat but now do so regularly, foods such as burdock root, Anasazi beans, various types of mushrooms, and wakame. I have since started to seek out these foods at higher end (and ethnic) markets that, I have noticed, once never carried these items but now do. When ingredients catch on with consumers, groceries respond. It's a reminder that grocery stores pay very close attention to consumer choices, which they carefully track. Get enough people to start asking for more promiscuous options at any grocery store and you will almost certainly see quick results. Even in East Texas.

—Make eating more nutrient dense foods a daily priority as well. Even within the limited range of options in front of us today there are genuine choices available for us to push our diets in the direction of greater nutrient density. Nutritional information can be notoriously shifty, but basic information about which foods contain which nutrients and in what amounts is abundantly available and generally trustworthy. At the least, we know blueberries and nuts and high-cocoa chocolate are better than chips and dips and salsa. As we seek nutrient density, it's important to allow concern for micronutrients to be our guide to eating, rather than concern for protein—which is, really, nothing more than an agribusiness trope that we've bought into all too easily. By eating a wide range of mostly plants that are nutrient dense, supplemented with small amounts of meat from non-domesticated animals, our protein needs will be more than met. Today, Americans actually get too much protein and, as we have seen, not enough micronutrients

—Eat meals out of bowls rather than off plates. Eating out of bowls encourages more creative combinations of more ingredients than the usual plate arrangement allows. For better or worse, the restaurants and chefs that have pioneered this trend have called these meals "hippie bowls." My favorite example of the humble but beautifully diversified hippie bowl comes from the elite and homogenous enclave of Cambridge, Massachusetts. Order a bowl called The Alchemist (my favorite) at Life Alive and you can get, in one sitting, sweet corn, carrots, ginger, kale, tofu, legumes, quinoa, sun-sprouts, and sunflower seeds. This template—whole grain, vegetables and nuts, dressing—has endless possibilities in terms of diversification and nutrient density. Add crunchy crickets, fried mealworms, and some seaweed and one is truly approaching the kind of promiscuity we should be envisioning for every meal we eat. Bowls also include soups, and soups, when done right, are complete meals—ones that can also be made in large quantities and saved for later consumption.

—Whenever possible prepare your own meals. Doing so is, of course, moderately time consuming, but do note that bowl-based meals can be made quickly and, as with soup, in large quantities to be eaten in the days ahead. Do not hesitate to experiment with various combinations of ingredients, as well as with when to eat certain foods. My experience has shown, for example, that there is nothing that hits the morning's empty stomach more satisfyingly than the salty broth of seaweed soup that Larch Hanson taught me to make. Remember that virtually everything we know and believe about food—what we eat, when we eat, how we eat—was made up by someone else, and it was made up to serve an end that may or may not be relevant to our own experience. This fact does not necessarily make our rules wrong, but it does make everything about food arbitrary and, therefore, capable of being changed.

—Relatedly, and finally, avoid restaurants. Be they fast-food places, mid-level Chili's-type establishments, or fancier venues, restaurants—which are widely heralded as luxuries—embody the absolute worst elements of today's food system. They make it too easy to leave our home kitchens, waste more food than home kitchens, directly support agribusiness, prepare meals that sometimes look healthy but are replete with hidden fat and sodium, encourage overeating, serve as venues of class distinction, rarely push the limits of promiscuity, and—this is more true for the farm-to-table places—promote a false sense of eco-correct dining. There is no eco-correct restaurant dining, at least when it comes to conventional restaurants. To the extent that we can, we should reserve our dining out dollars for the kinds of eating venues that, in so far as they depart from the restaurant norm, provide food that supports promiscuity, affordability, and family-style dining while minimizing waste and classist pomp. Food trucks have the potential to enact these ideals on a broad scale. A food truck serving a hippie bowl with

fifteen healthy ingredients in it—this is what I'm envisioning all
of us eating as routine meals of the future.

More than anything else, remember this: We are not, contrary to what
the old saying insists, what we eat. Given the agricultural system we have
inherited, and given the food options currently around us, we are better
than what we eat. We are more complicated and thoughtful than what
we eat. We contain multitudes that our food refuses to honor. The narrow but abundant food pageantry that's paraded before us is an insult to
our health, the health of the environment, and the welfare of animals.
When it's possible for a person concerned with eating promiscuously (as
it's defined in this book) to walk into a convenience store and, aside from
beer and nuts, not find a single item that's consistent with his dietary ideals, then you know at least two things are true: a) That person's culinary
standards are in the right place; b) Something has gone badly wrong
with the way we feed ourselves.

This situation, despite the constant rhetoric of choice and abundance that infuses our dialogues over food, has been foisted on us. History chose it for us. But, in the present, the agribusiness machine that
provides our food also chooses it for us, and it does so without regard
for our health or the ideals we ask food to uphold and embody. We have
said yes too long to the status quo. We have done so because the status
quo has been normalized to the point that we cannot imagine starting
over. But we can start over. There are other ways to eat. It's time to tap
our inner bonobo, get food right, and work towards a food system that
allows everyone to eat promiscuously.

# Acknowledgments

TK